MW00682475

SEASONS OF LIFE

Designs for Reaping the Rewards of Autumn

Editors *Carol Shea*
Bruce Arant
Plans Editor *Tina Leyden*
Art Director *Sharon T. Potter*
Graphic Designers *Yen Gutowski*
Gloria Chavez
Illustrator *Heather Bettinger*
Rendering Colorization *Alva Louden*
Rendering Illustrators *Shawn Doherty*
Silvia Boyd
Perry Gauthier
George McDonald, dec.
Technical Adviser *Jody Marker*
Managing Editor *Kevin Blair*
Publisher *Dennis Brozak*
Associate Publisher *Linda Reimer*

SEASONS OF LIFE™
Designs for Reaping the Rewards of Autumn
is published by:
Design Basics Publications
11112 John Galt Blvd., Omaha, NE 68137
Web – www.designbasics.com
Email – dbi@synergy.net

Chief Executive Officer *Dennis Brozak*
President *Linda Reimer*
Director of Marketing *Kevin Blair*
Business Development *Paul Foresman*
Controller *Janie Murnane*

Text and Design © 1997 by Design Basics Inc.
All rights reserved.

No part of this publication may be reproduced in any form or by any means without prior written permission of the publisher.

Cover Photo: Plan #2408 Cordeaux
As seen on page 41

Builder: Lewis Builders Inc.
Photo by: Carl Saporiti

design basics inc. HOME PLAN DESIGN SERVICE

Library of Congress Number: 97-092483
ISBN: 0-9647658

One-Story home plans

1 1/2-Story home plans

1 1/2-Story home plans

Two-Story home plans

Duplex home plans

If life could be categorized by seasons, you could say that those who are empty-nesters would be moving into their autumn years.

Vastly different from their predecessors, the empty-nesters of today face an unprecedented range of opportunities and choices. For them, the changing of the seasons leaves them no longer engrossed in raising their children. They are, in a sense, starting over.

Autumn gives us vibrance in the changing colors of the trees and cool solace after long, hot summers – much like the empty- nest stage of life. Vastly different from their predecessors, the empty-nesters of today face an unprecedented range of opportunities and choices. For them, the changing of the seasons leaves them no longer engrossed in raising their children. They are, in a sense, starting over. Some are choosing to retire. Others are starting new careers. Whatever their choice, none are ready to idly sit by.

All across the country, their ranks continue to swell with the aging of the "Baby Boomer" generation (Statistics say 10,000 people turn 50 every day). The sheer size of their number leaves no doubt that their idea and beliefs will have a profound effect o many things in our society, one of whic being the homes they will live in.

Empty-nesters of toda are interested in living lif to the fullest. As a group they are better educate than their parents and mor likely than not to be married And while many of them ar once again living alone, it's fact that for many others, the nes is not always empty. Several face the reality o having to care for an elderly parent or a "boomerang" – an older child who' come back to live with them. And still others are stepping in to help care fo their grandchildren.

They are interested in outliving the age of their parents and as a result, a more active than ever. They are teaching aerobics, jogging and watching what the eat – even on their vacations. Studies tell us they are traveling more, golfin prodigiously and drinking diet Coke. In short, it is clear they are actively enjoyin their post-parenting years.

Today's empty-nesters generally fall into one of two categories: th "Matures" age 55 and up and the "Boomers" age 45 - 55 years old. While the lifestage as "empty-nesters" is the same, their reactions and values are often di ferent, based on their experiences early in life. The Matures grew up in times of personal sacrifice and war. Their attitudes, therefore, tend to be conservative and disciplined. They view vacations and retirement as rewards for their years of hard work. The Boomers, on the other hand, grew up in times of economic prosperity, helping them formulate high expectations in life. "Boomers tend to have an attitude of ent tlement created by their presumption of economic growth according to Inc. magazine. And what these t groups of empty-nesters desire in housing is reflec ed in these attitudes.

It would appear that what they want in a hor would be different, but surprisingly, the opposite true. It's only their attitudes of "reward" a

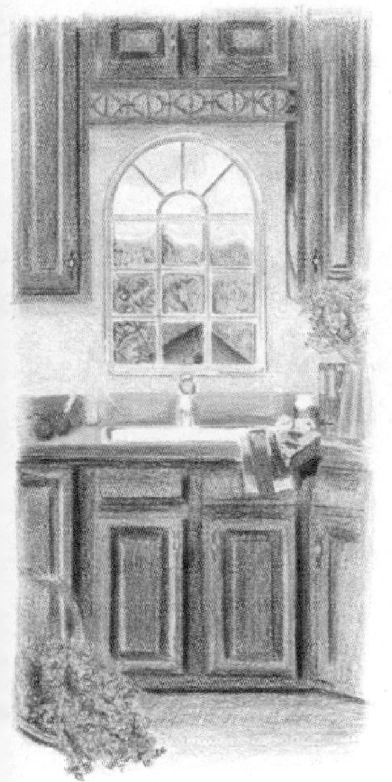

"entitlement" that set them apart. Both groups want a home that reflects their desire for natural beauty – mature landscaping and views that they can enjoy from within their homes. This corresponds with their desire for plenty of windows to appreciate the beauty of the outdoors. Additionally, an abundance of windows provides a great source of natural light which today's empty-nesters also crave. A case in point is illustrated by builder Russ Sweetman of Centerville, OH. As a builder of custom homes, Sweetman satisfies his empty-nester buyers by including sunrooms and elaborate kitchen windows as beautiful as the picture windows traditionally found in formal or family rooms.

Home offices are also important to today's empty-nester, many of whom, as they approach retirement, are choosing to continue to work from their homes. Others look to the home itself to provide another source of income. Many are purchasing multifamily homes, such as duplexes, and renting out the other living spaces to supplement their income.

Both groups of empty nesters are interested in homes that might be thought of as "jewel boxes" – homes that are modest in square footage and packed with amenities. They want security systems or gated communities for safety. They want volume ceilings for a sense of openness and built-in bookcases to shelve their favorite reading material. They prefer hobby rooms, three-car garages and pampering master suites.

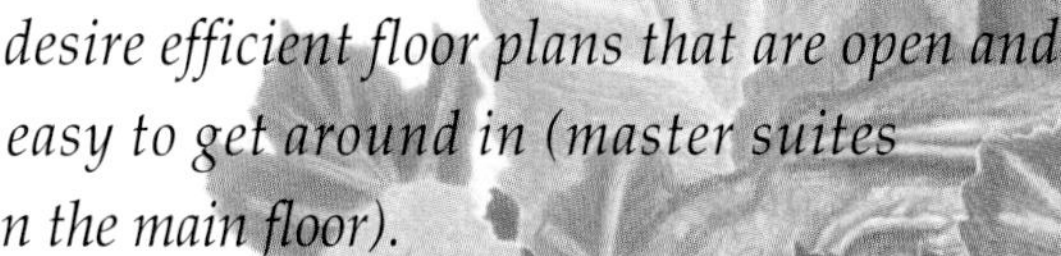

Recreational activities are also very important to the empty-nester, not only for personal enjoyment, but also for health-related reasons. Therefore, accessibility to golf courses, biking/hiking trails, and health clubs is essential.

Empty-nesters wish to spend less time upkeeping their home, translating into their desire for low-maintenance homes, such as those with brick exteriors or permanent clad siding. They desire efficient floor plans that are open and easy to get around in (master suites on the main floor).

All of these preferences in home design are reflected in the following 100 designs. We at Design Basics believe that each of them uniquely benefits the empty-nester. The plans feature a wide variety of amenities and square footages, and each can be customized to adapt to the special needs and desires of most any buyer.

Entering into a new "Season" of life, today's empty-nesters bring their unique characteristics into a wide realm of opportunities that lie ahead. The home they choose to build will be one of the most exciting opportunities of all. ◆

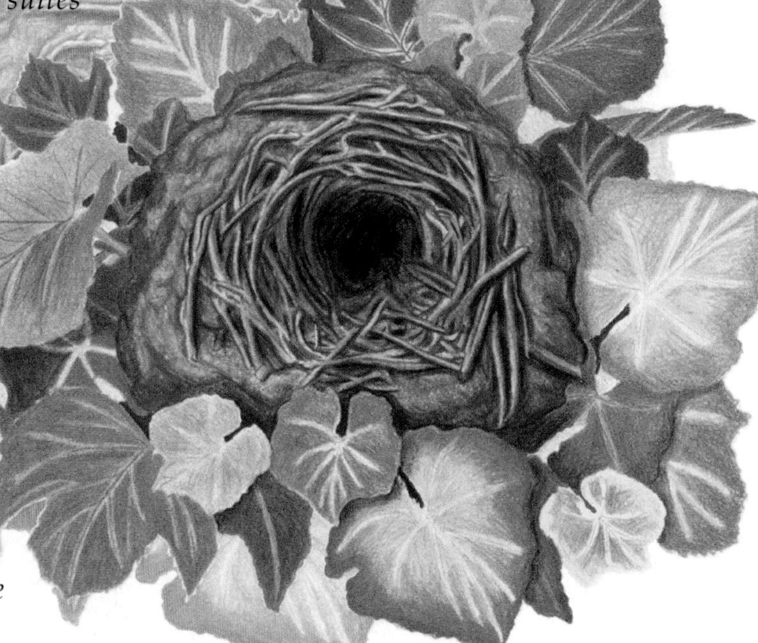

My middle son recently moved back home to live in our basement and return to college. Just having him around again has caused me to reflect on the years we had the children with us and this house that bore the brunt of our life. This house is different now – all hardwood floors, a few shaker antiques and sparse, eclectic decor. This is the house of our now professional, post-children lives. It's just the two of us again, getting groceries only occasionally, working late into the night and being faithful to our local health club. It's a far cry from this home's fully carpeted, country-craft past. And even further from its shag carpet and wall mural days. We have settled into our professional lives knowing the full and rich life we had with our children. And we draw upon those hectic, fruitful years, relishing the memories for a good laugh and a sense of pride. It is unfortunate that I hardly ever take this time to look back. My direction in life has always been focused on the future. And because of this, I wonder if those whom I've been acquainted with for some time, can ever really know me, without knowing my past, my story in this home.

Step into my home where, in 1977, my husband and I dropped our suitcases and boxes filled with tennis racquets and ceramic dishes.

If you want to know me – I would mentally say to them - if you wish to see where I've been, where I am going, step into my house. Step into my home where, in 1977, my husband and I dropped our suitcases and boxes filled with tennis racquets and ceramic dishes. Envision the little green house we left on 4th Street to be the third owners of a bi-level in the southwest part of town. I'd had our four children by that time – the youngest just three months old. Step into my home and see that it was here we paused to raise them and nurture them into adulthood.

Walk into my family room, a 20′x 20′ monster that's the first to greet you when you walk in the door. It showcased our wall murals and was later wallpapered in country print. Walk with me the many times I stepped over bodies on my way to work the morning after a sleepover. Or the times I came home to our modular furniture constructed into the forts of mighty warlords.

cont'd on next page

Creighton

#28A-4208 Plan Price $535

Total Square Feet: 2057 Sq. Ft.

An angled garage makes the home useable on a narrower lot.

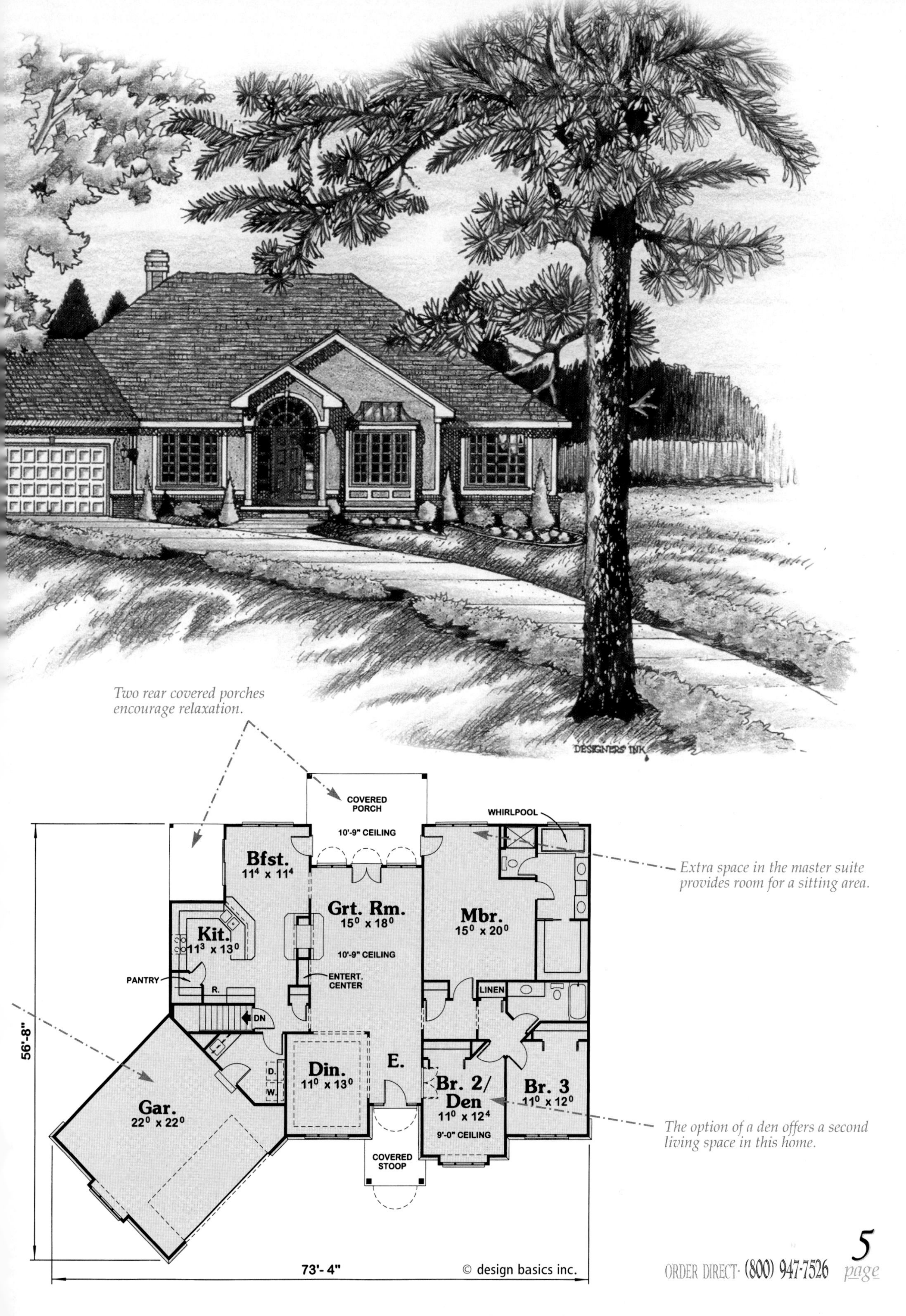
DESIGNERS' INK
Two rear covered porches encourage relaxation.
COVERED PORCH
10'-9" CEILING
WHIRLPOOL
Bfst.
11⁴ x 11⁴
Grt. Rm.
15⁰ x 18⁰
10'-9" CEILING
ENTERT. CENTER
Kit.
11³ x 13⁰
PANTRY
R.
DN
Mbr.
15⁰ x 20⁰
LINEN
Extra space in the master suite provides room for a sitting area.
56'-8"
Din.
11⁰ x 13⁰
E.
D.
W.
Br. 2/ Den
11⁰ x 12⁴
9'-0" CEILING
Br. 3
11⁰ x 12⁰
The option of a den offers a second living space in this home.
Gar.
22⁰ x 22⁰
COVERED STOOP
73'- 4"
© design basics inc.

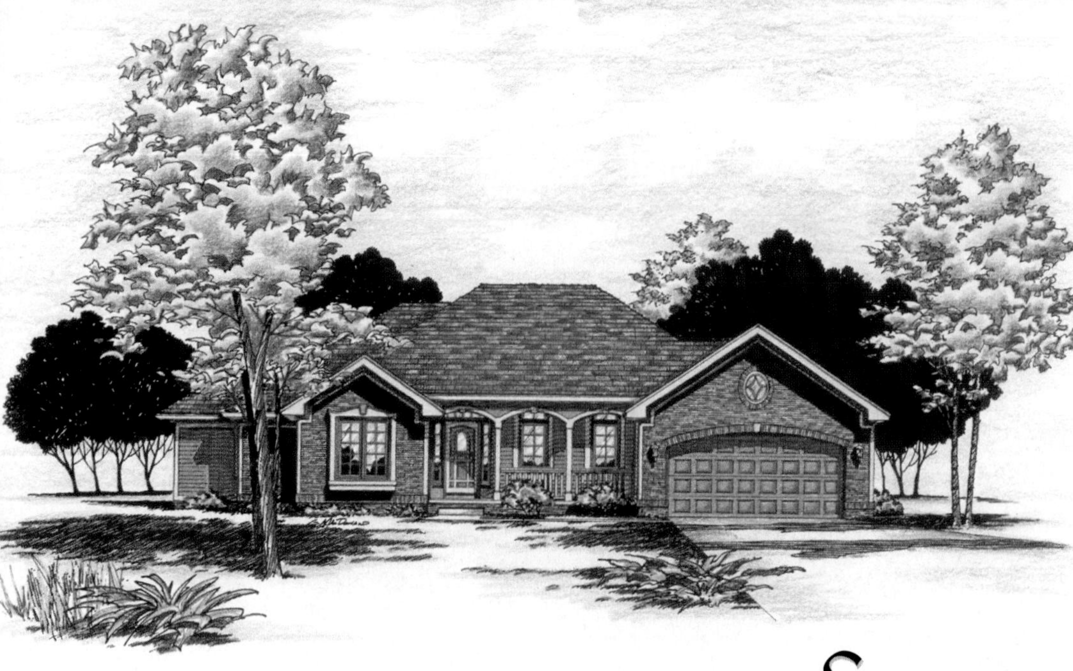

Surrey

Total Square Feet: 1948 Sq. Ft.

#28A-2384 Plan Price $525

First impressions of expansive space come from uninhibited views of the open dining room and great room.

The generous master suite offers a roomy bath area with his and her lavs and a large corner whirlpool tub.

Entertaining is enhanced by a wet bar between the breakfast area and great room.

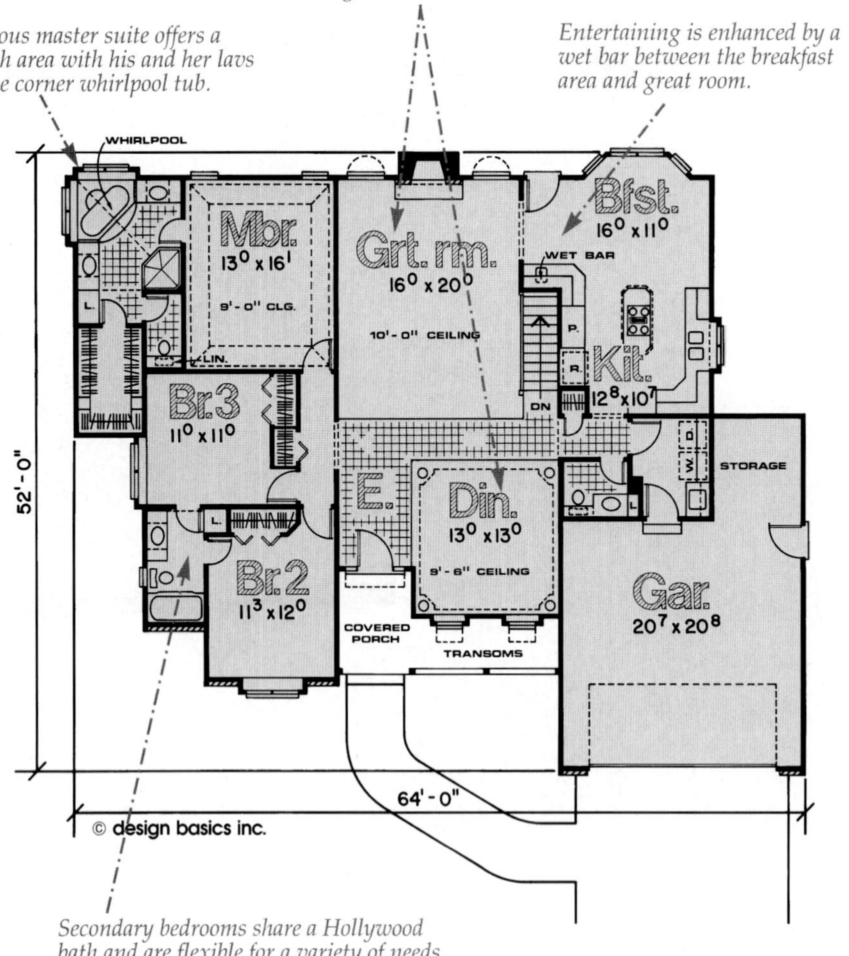

Secondary bedrooms share a Hollywood bath and are flexible for a variety of needs.

You must see the 6:00 a.m. birthday parties I threw for the kids – the dining room embellished with balloons and ribbon followed by a birthday breakfast.

To know me you must walk up the four steps to where my living room, dining room, kitchen and main bedrooms are. You must see the 6:00 a.m. birthday parties I threw for the kids – the dining room embellished with balloons and ribbon followed by a birthday breakfast. And the kitchen where I made elaborate holiday dinners, and like the Betty Crocker's of the world, froze portions of casseroles for the upcoming week. You must walk into my sons' bedroom where hours upon hours of enjoyment was infused in a wall-mounted basketball hoop and free throw line taped on the floor. And smell the lingering waft of acrylic in my bedroom-turned-den, where I painted crafts long into the night for my home business. Walk the backyard with worn patches from baseball and football games and countless water slide afternoons. And experience the garage where a former owner was rumored to have passed on – and was for years shunned by my children for fear of his ghost. And

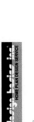

cont'd on next page

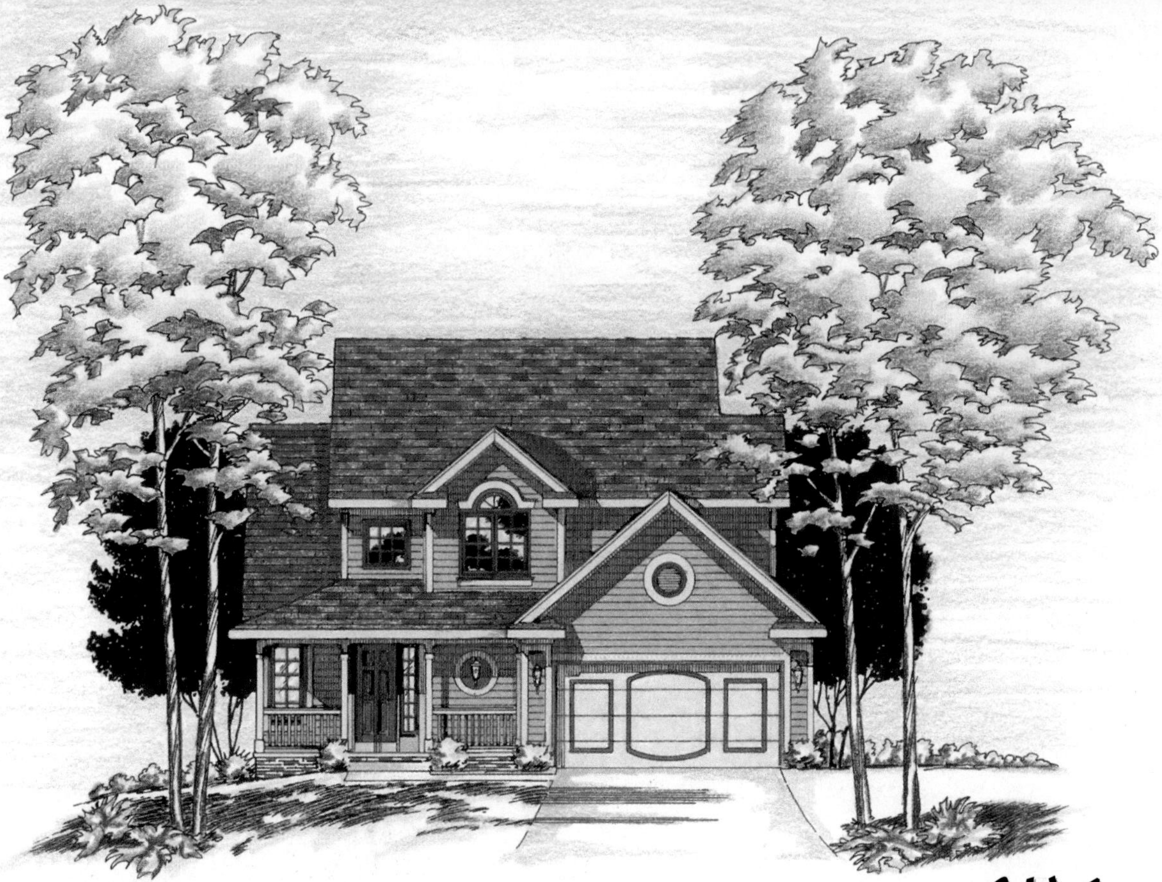

Webster

#28A-3582 Plan Price $495

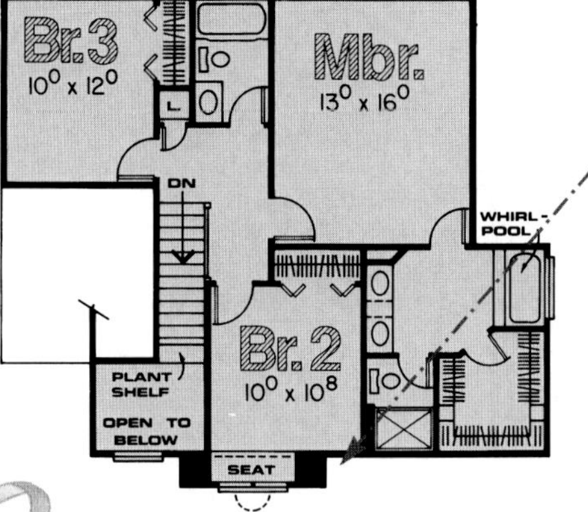

A window seat in bedroom #2 enhances the room's character, whether it's used as originally intended, or put to use as a hobby or sewing room.

The sunlit family room is situated for privacy and openly flows into the breakfast area.

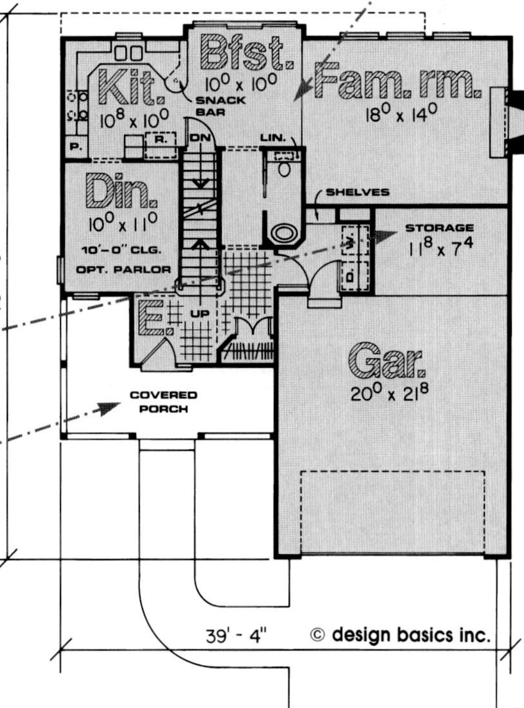

A generous storage area adds practical space to the garage.

The wrap-around country porch gives an added sense of "welcome" to the front of this home.

Main Floor:	*866 Sq. Ft.*
Second Floor:	*785 Sq. Ft.*
Total Square Feet:	*1651 Sq. Ft.*

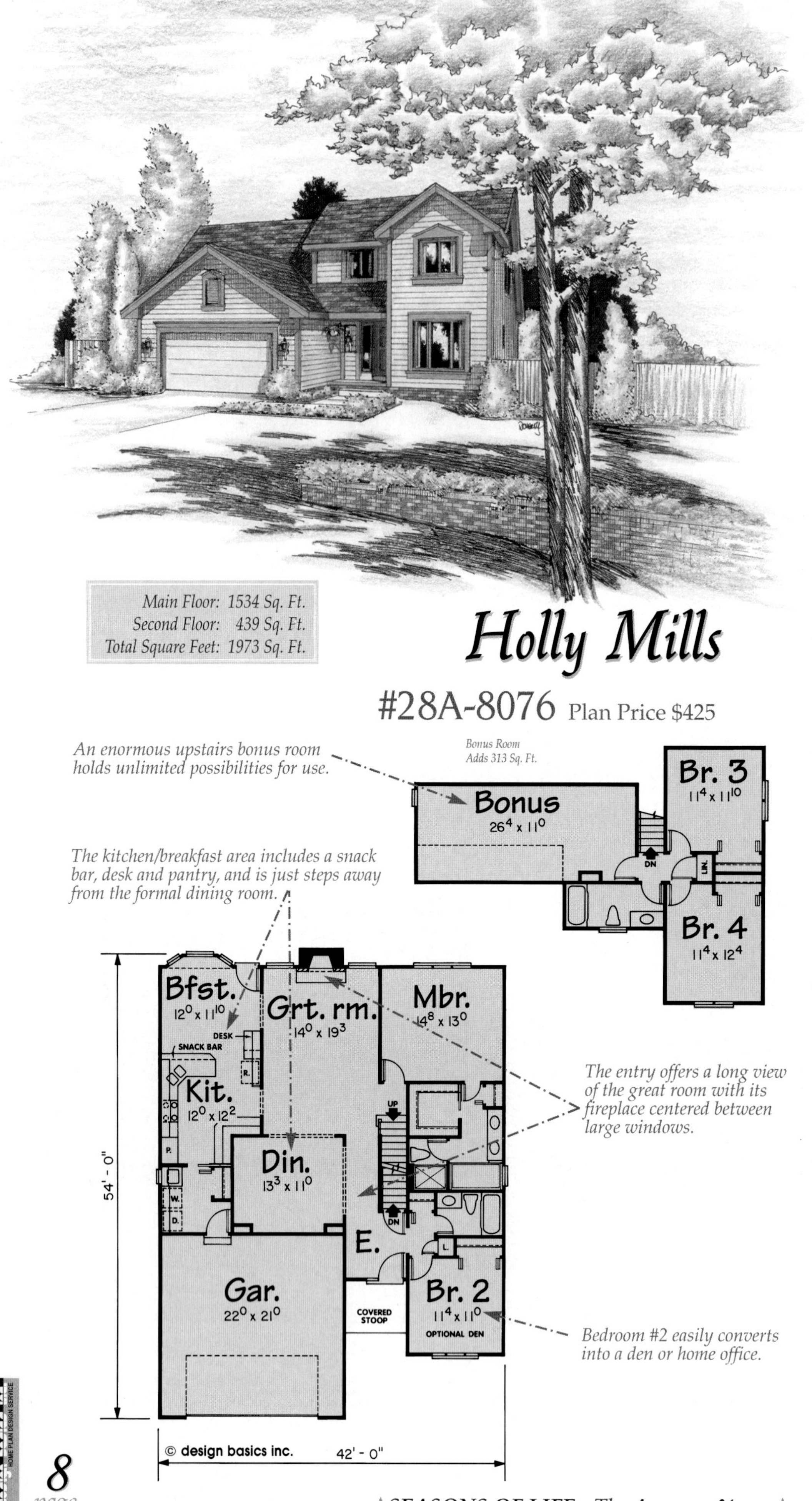

Main Floor: 1534 Sq. Ft.
Second Floor: 439 Sq. Ft.
Total Square Feet: 1973 Sq. Ft.

Holly Mills

#28A-8076 Plan Price $425

An enormous upstairs bonus room holds unlimited possibilities for use.

The kitchen/breakfast area includes a snack bar, desk and pantry, and is just steps away from the formal dining room.

The entry offers a long view of the great room with its fireplace centered between large windows.

Bedroom #2 easily converts into a den or home office.

You must walk into my son's bedroom where hours upon hours of enjoyment was infused in a wall-mounted basketball hoop and free throw line taped on the floor.

that not once over these 20 years, to our regret, has he shown up. You must look past our polished home of today and comprehend the messy, inconsistencies of its past. You must experience, as we did, the way in which it sheltered our anxieties and exalted our joys. You must see my house and simultaneously see my family's formative years resting deep in its character.

It is then you'll discover that all of this is only significant because of where it has brought me today. You'll discover the journey I've taken and that knowing me fully, I'll rarely look back on it all. You will know that I'll inevitably find new ways to decorate my home and new ways to celebrate birthday parties. And that in leaving this house behind, I'll find a new place to call home. ◆

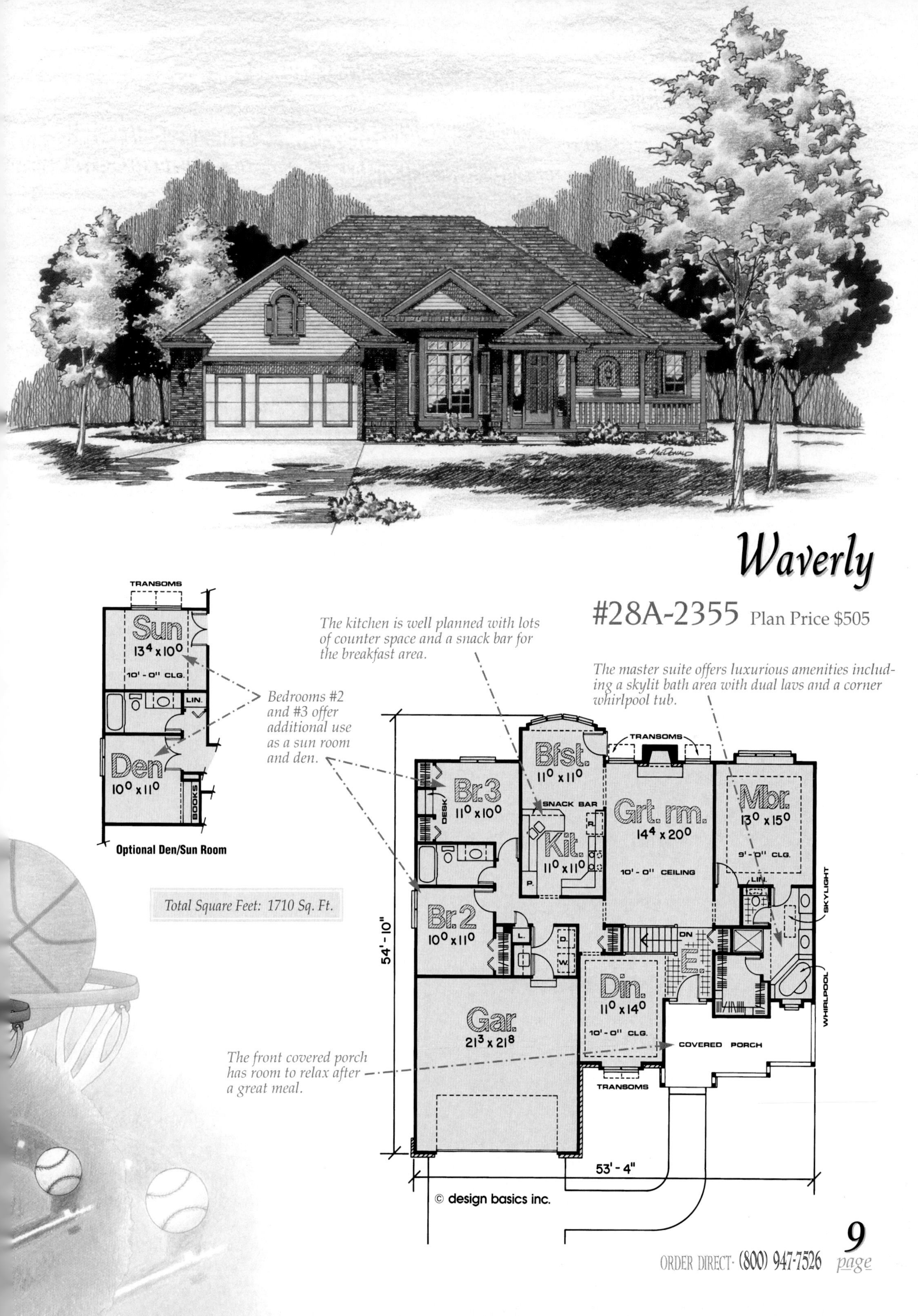

Waverly

#28A-2355 Plan Price $505

The kitchen is well planned with lots of counter space and a snack bar for the breakfast area.

The master suite offers luxurious amenities including a skylit bath area with dual lavs and a corner whirlpool tub.

Bedrooms #2 and #3 offer additional use as a sun room and den.

The front covered porch has room to relax after a great meal.

Total Square Feet: 1710 Sq. Ft.

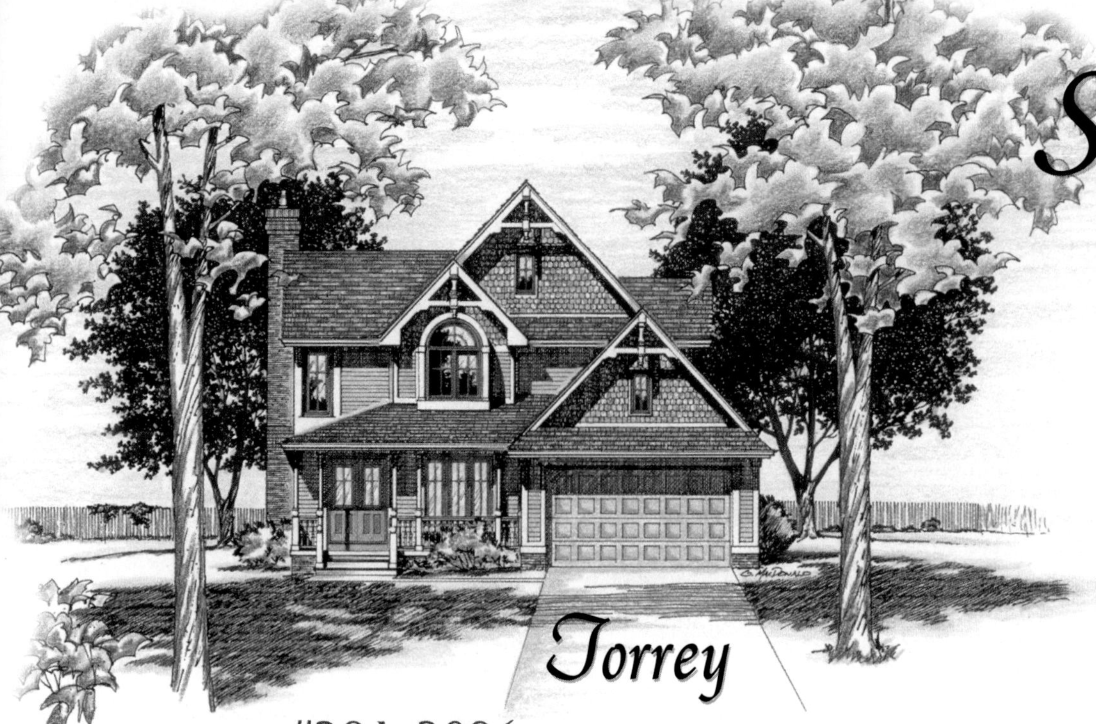

Torrey

#28A-3096 Plan Price $505

Main Floor: 905 Sq. Ft.
Second Floor: 863 Sq. Ft.
Total Square Feet: 1768 Sq. Ft.

Many windows line the rear of the home, offering excellent views.

The island kitchen with snack bar features plenty of light from the breakfast area and an angled window above the sink.

A window seat brings a sense of nostalgia to the front entry.

© design basics inc.

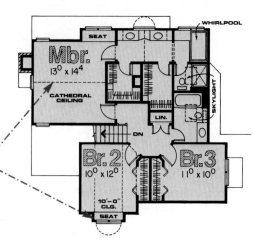

Volume ceilings and window seats add a sense of spaciousness to bedroom #2 and the master suite.

SITUATION

There's nothing I like better than to sit outside and appreciate the things surrounding me. I'm done with the rat race. I need a place with no TV. No office work or computers. Just me, a cup of tea and a comfortable chair. The kind of place that makes me remember the kids. The kind of place that makes me want to take some time off with my husband. Yes, I need a porch. . .

SOLUTION

Deep porches wrap both the front and rear of the Torrey (❶, at left). Furnishing the two porches as outdoor living spaces leaves the choice of enjoying either area no matter the time of day. A wonderful place to relax in the Orchard is its rear covered porch, (❷, at right and interior view). With room for a table and chairs, it's the perfect place to retire to with guests.

design basics inc. HOME PLAN DESIGN SERVICE

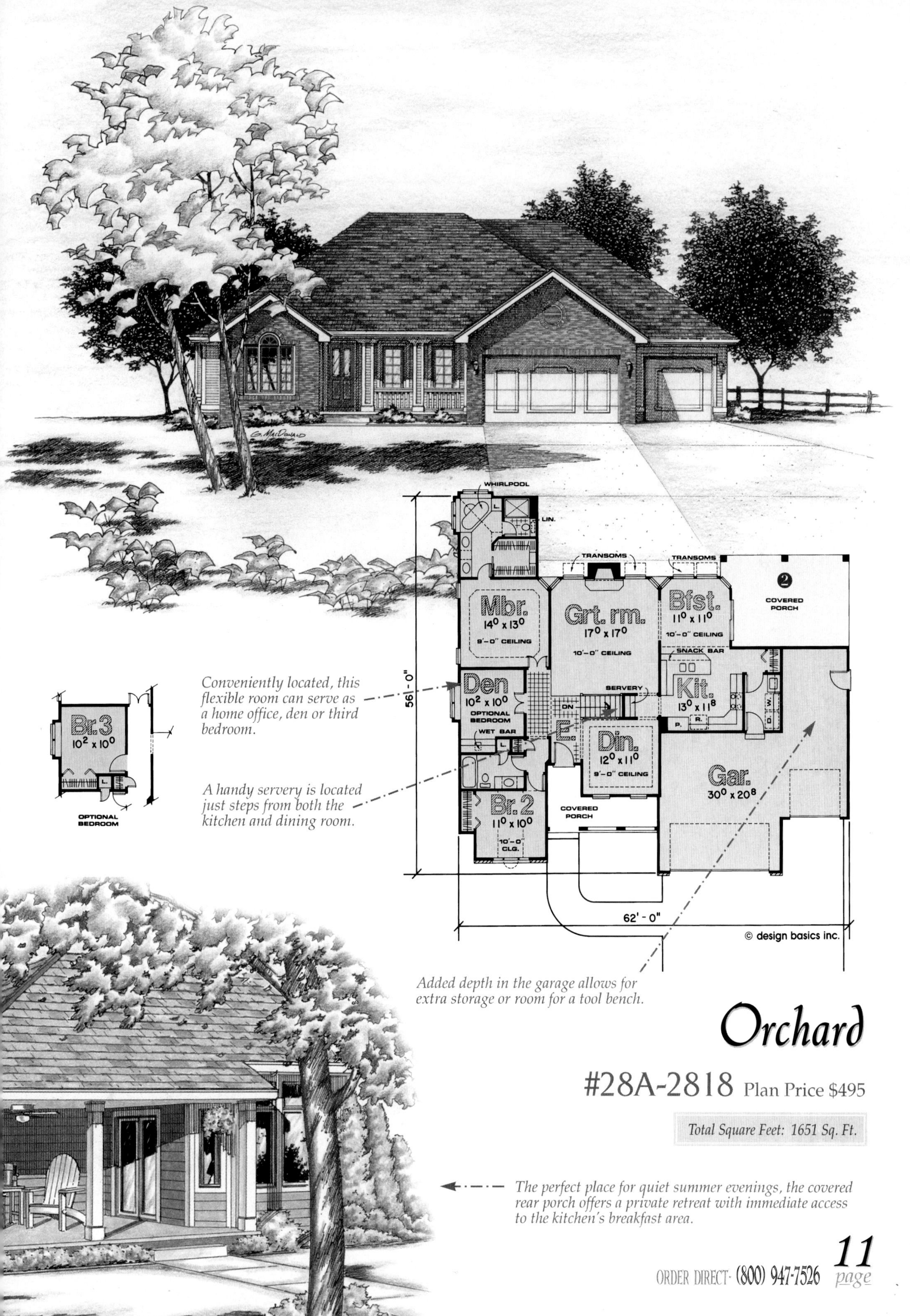

Conveniently located, this flexible room can serve as a home office, den or third bedroom.

A handy servery is located just steps from both the kitchen and dining room.

Added depth in the garage allows for extra storage or room for a tool bench.

Orchard

#28A-2818 Plan Price $495

Total Square Feet: 1651 Sq. Ft.

The perfect place for quiet summer evenings, the covered rear porch offers a private retreat with immediate access to the kitchen's breakfast area.

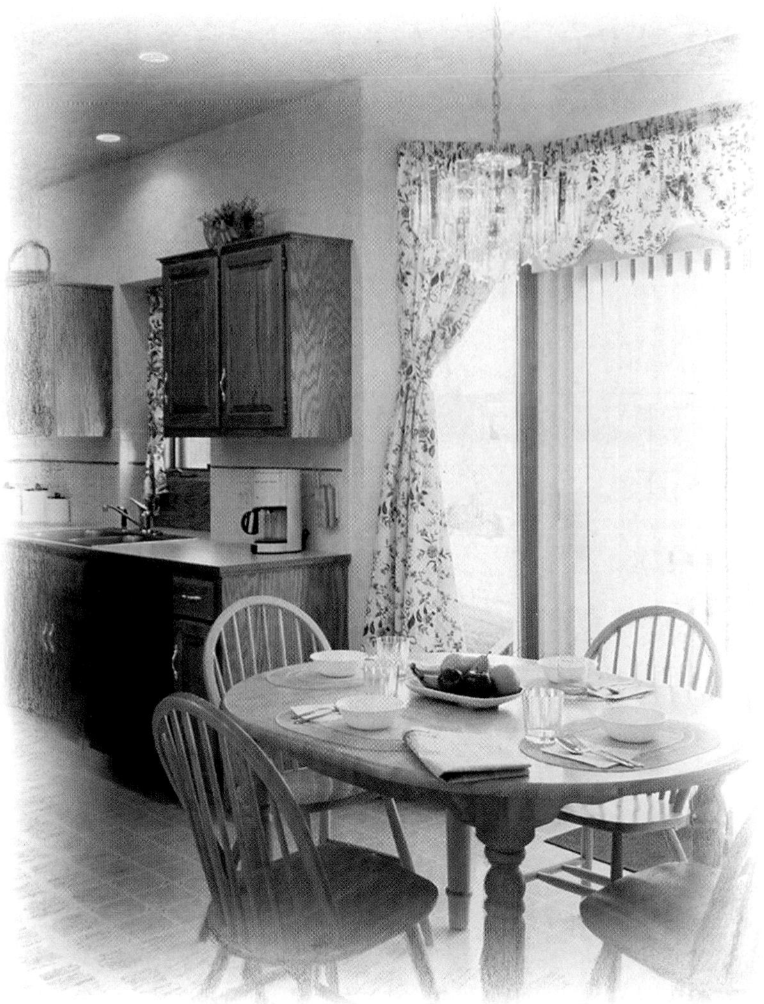

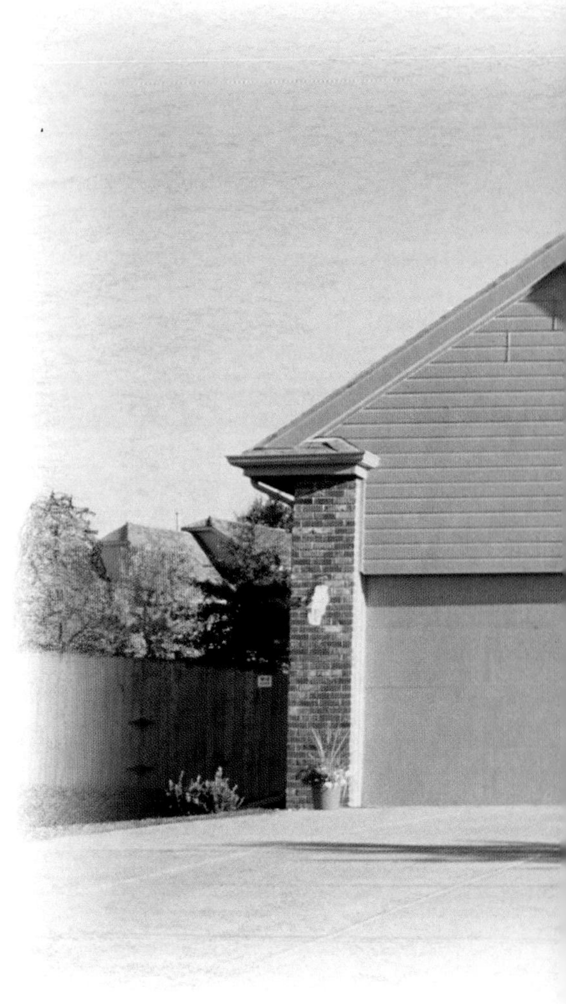

ABOVE LEFT: A comfortable breakfast area is strategically located between the kitchen and great room.

RIGHT: The focus in the great room centers on a fireplace flanked between tall windows.

BUILT BY: MAJESTIC HOMES
PHOTO BY: JEFF BEBEE

The home in these photographs may be altered from the original plan.

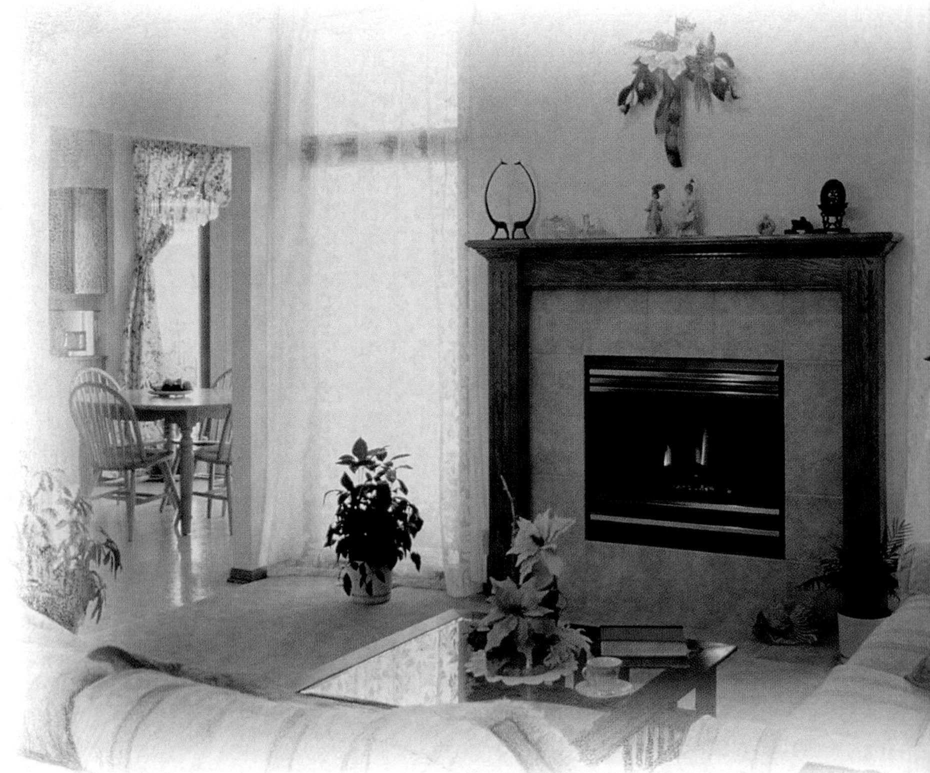

Total Square Feet: 1496 Sq. Ft.

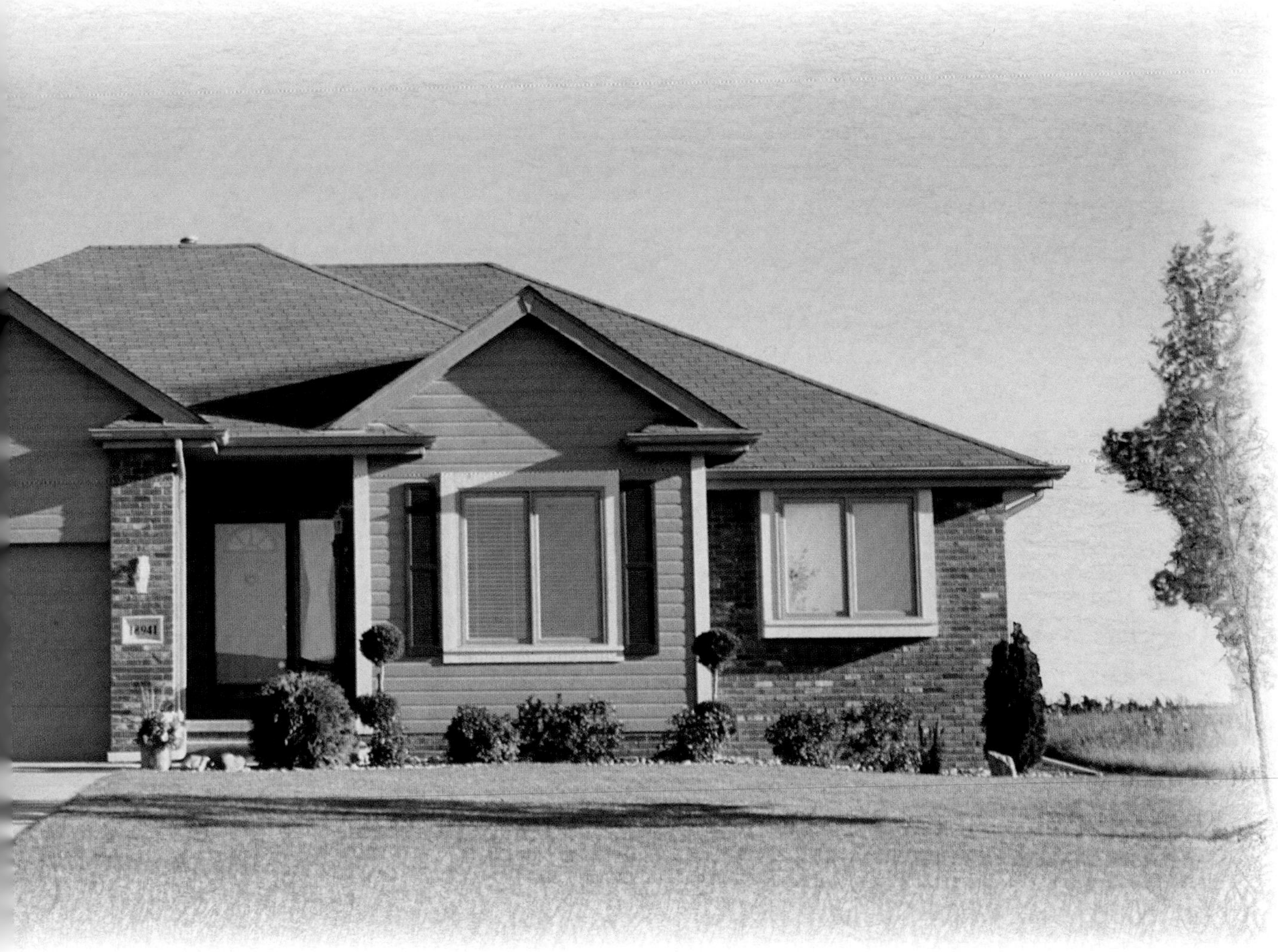

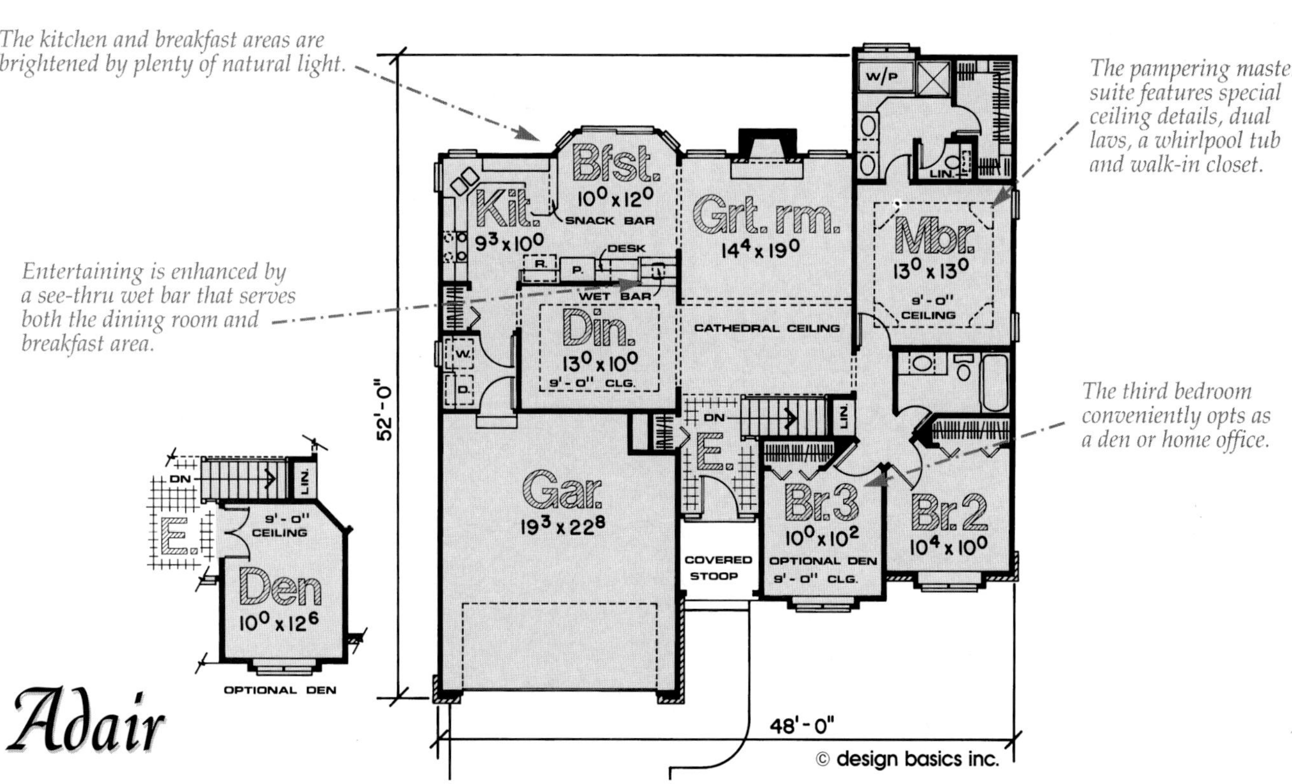

The kitchen and breakfast areas are brightened by plenty of natural light.

Entertaining is enhanced by a see-thru wet bar that serves both the dining room and breakfast area.

The pampering master suite features special ceiling details, dual lavs, a whirlpool tub and walk-in closet.

The third bedroom conveniently opts as a den or home office.

Adair

#28A-2300 Plan Price $475

SITUATION

Since my father passed away, we've really felt the need to have my mother live with us. She can still function quite well on her own, but as she gets older, we'd feel better if we could provide her with the option of living with us. We've been thinking of moving into a new home anyway, so what we really need is a design that provides private living quarters for her. . .

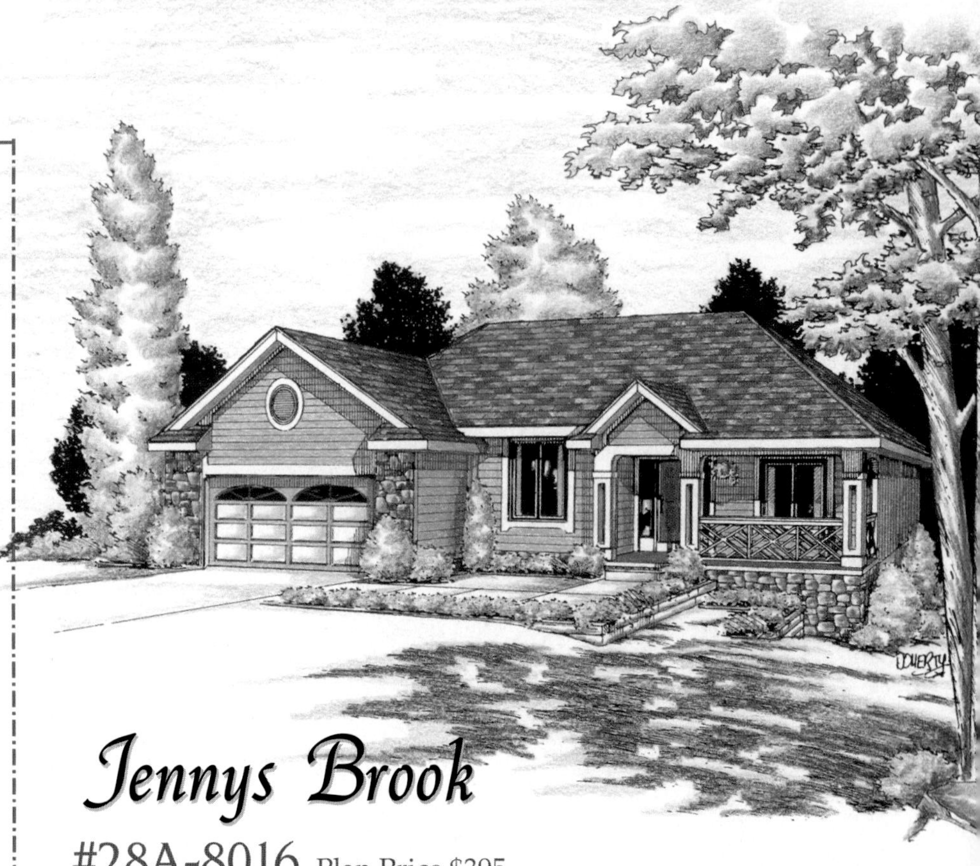

Jennys Brook

#28A-8016 Plan Price $395

Total Square Feet: 1691 Sq. Ft.

SOLUTION

The Fairway features several options for live-in relatives. It's finished basement has the advantage of a totally separated living area with a separate entrance (❶, at far right). And just inside the entry, the den has its own bath and could be converted into a bedroom. Separate bedroom wings in the Jennys Brook offers the option of integrating the two secondary bedrooms into private living space for a live-in relative (❷, at right).

The well-lit breakfast area provides a pleasant view of nature through bayed windows.

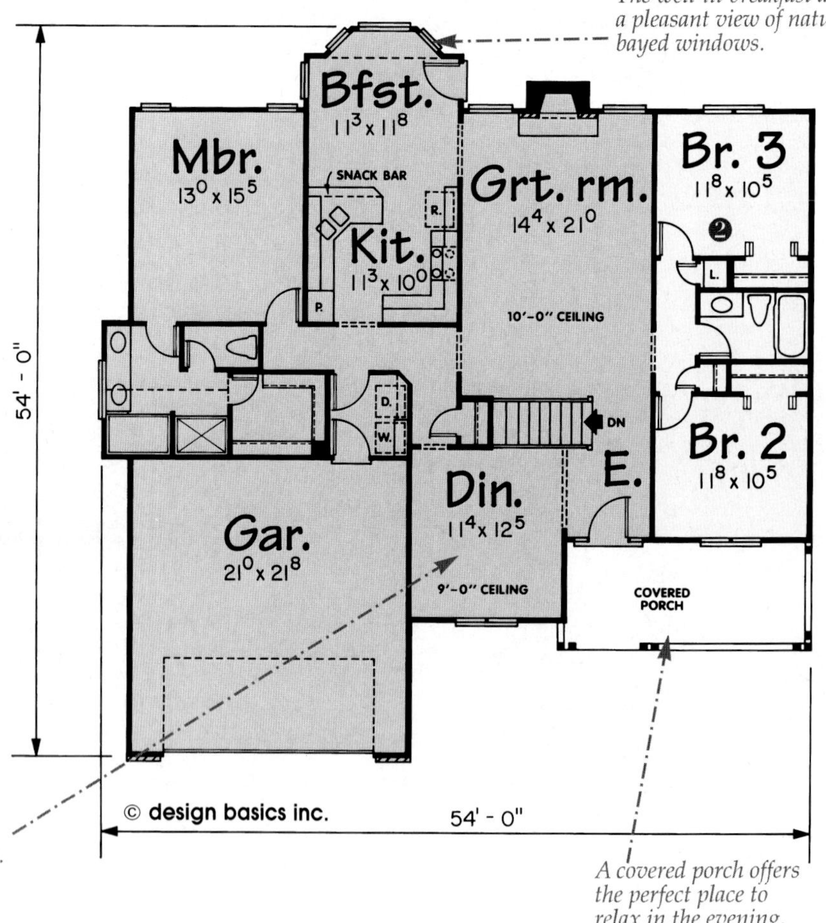

A dining room offers a memorable place for the family to eat during the holidays.

A covered porch offers the perfect place to relax in the evening.

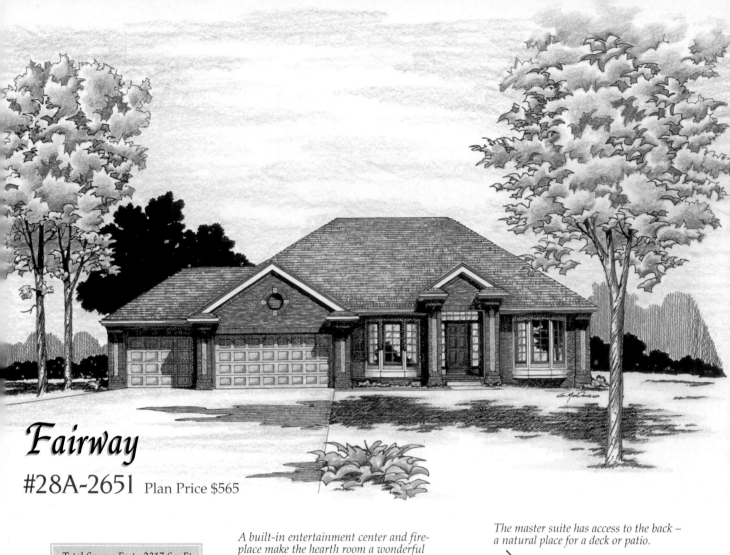

Fairway

#28A-2651 Plan Price $565

Total Square Feet: 2317 Sq. Ft.

A built-in entertainment center and fireplace make the hearth room a wonderful place to relax in.

The master suite has access to the back – a natural place for a deck or patio.

The large kitchen features an island cooktop to easily prepare elaborate dinners.

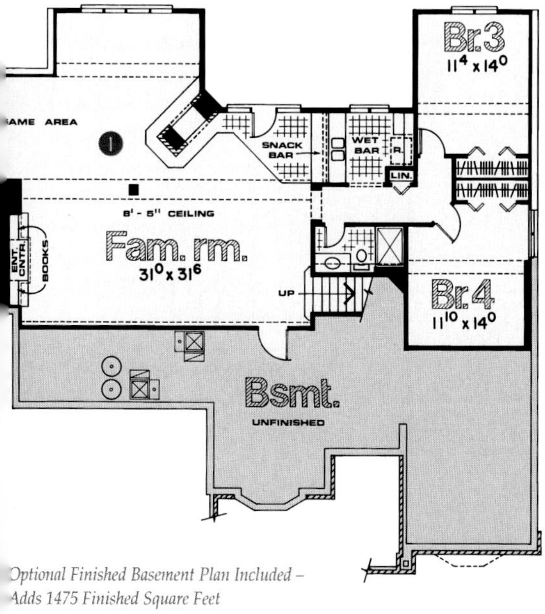

GAME AREA
SNACK BAR
WET BAR
R.
LIN.
8' - 5" CEILING
Fam. rm.
31⁰ x 31⁶
ENT. CNTR.
BOOKS
UP
Br.3
11⁴ x 14⁰
Br.4
11¹⁰ x 14⁰
Bsmt.
UNFINISHED

Optional Finished Basement Plan Included – Adds 1475 Finished Square Feet

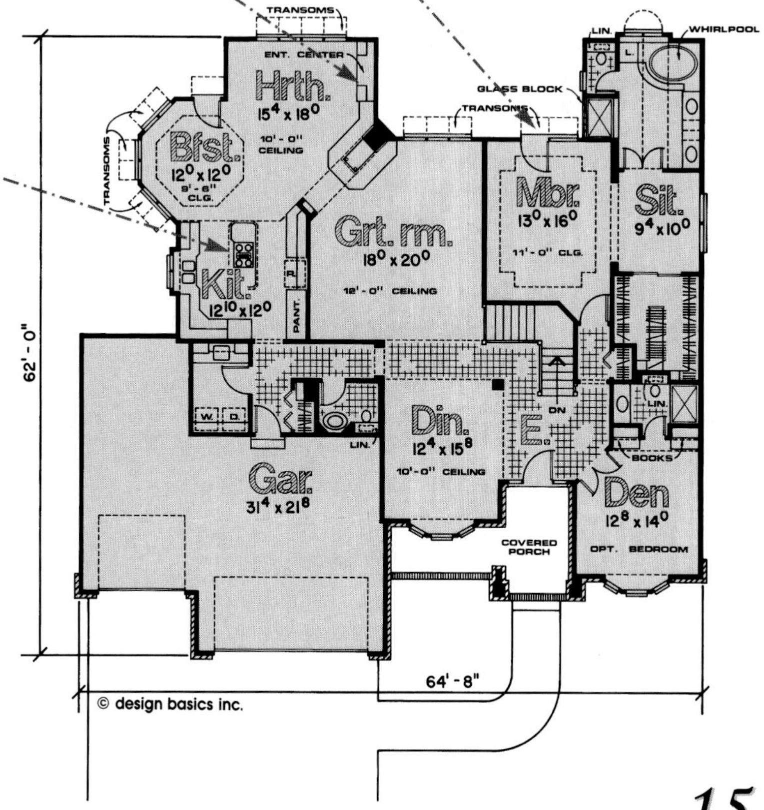

TRANSOMS
ENT. CENTER
Hrth.
15⁴ x 18⁰
10' - 0" CEILING
Bfst.
12⁰ x 12⁰
9' - 6" CLG.
TRANSOMS
Kit.
12¹⁰ x 12⁰
PANT.
R
Grt. rm.
18⁰ x 20⁰
12' - 0" CEILING
GLASS BLOCK
TRANSOMS
LIN.
WHIRLPOOL
Mbr.
13⁰ x 16⁰
11' - 0" CLG.
Sit.
9⁴ x 10⁰
W. D.
LIN.
Din.
12⁴ x 15⁸
10' - 0" CEILING
DN
E.
LIN.
BOOKS
Den
12⁸ x 14⁰
OPT. BEDROOM
Gar.
31⁴ x 21⁸
COVERED PORCH
62' - 0"
64' - 8"
© design basics inc.

HOME OFFICE SPACE . . . *Today's working professionals don't confine themselves solely to the office. Therefore, today's home plans need flexible rooms that can serve a variety of functions, such as that of a home office. The following plans offer this option through a variety of unique and well-planned designs.*

OPEN TO THE ENTRY

Main Floor: 1701 Sq. Ft.
Second Floor: 639 Sq. Ft.
Total Square Feet: 2340 Sq. Ft.

Ambrose

#28A-2701 Plan Price $565

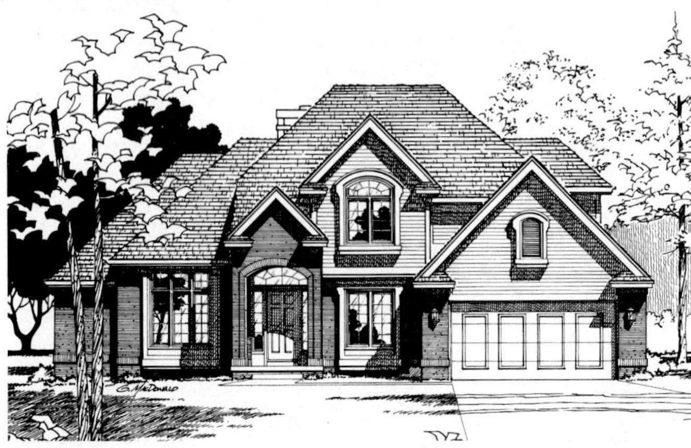

A skylight illuminates the master bath featuring an oval whirlpool and long walk-in closet.

The spacious kitchen and breakfast area welcome guests from the impressive great room.

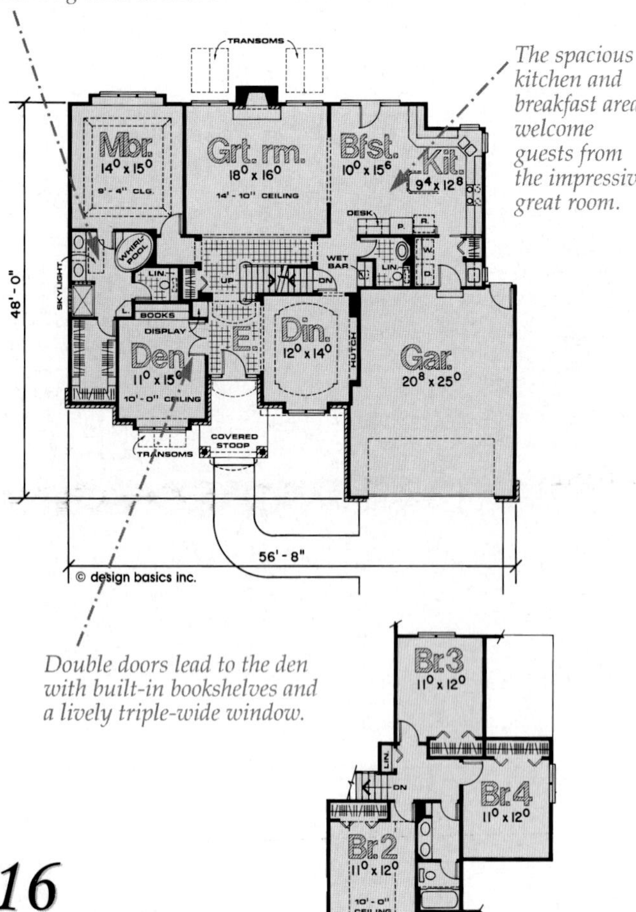

Double doors lead to the den with built-in bookshelves and a lively triple-wide window.

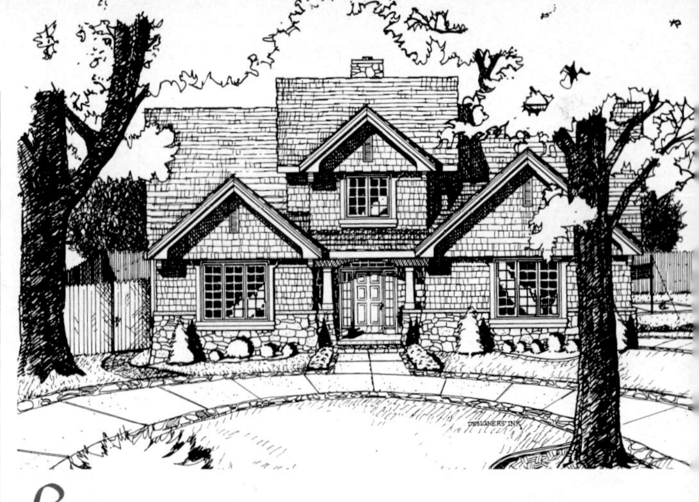

LOFTY ALTERNATIVES

Main Floor: 1640 Sq. Ft.
Second Floor: 711 Sq. Ft.
Total Square Feet: 2351 Sq. Ft.

Kenneth

#28A-4082 Plan Price $565

A rear staircase is convenient to the family area.

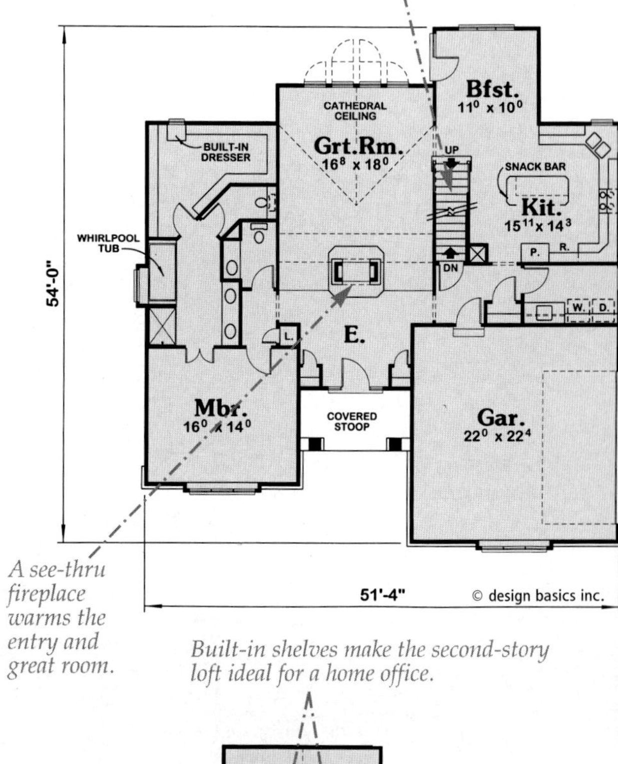

A see-thru fireplace warms the entry and great room.

Built-in shelves make the second-story loft ideal for a home office.

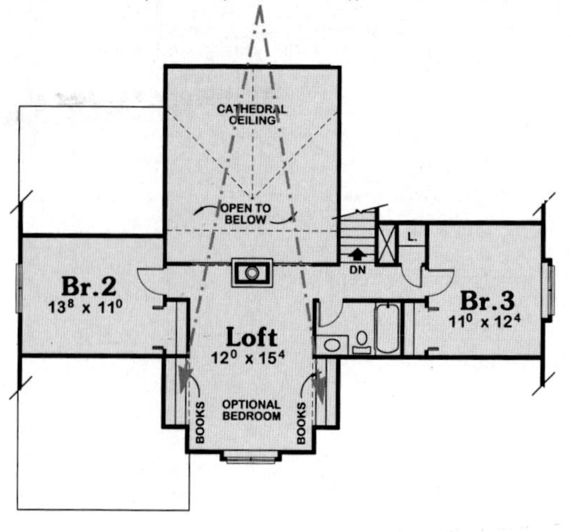

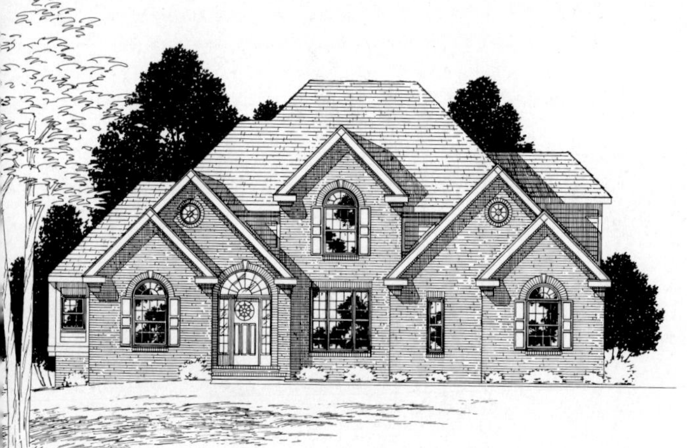

OUT-OF-THE-WAY WORKSPACE

Main Floor: 2000 Sq. Ft.
Second Floor: 764 Sq. Ft.
Total Square Feet: 2764 Sq. Ft.

MacCready

#28A-3484 Plan Price $605

An office between the kitchen and garage provides numerous benefits for the work-at-home professional.

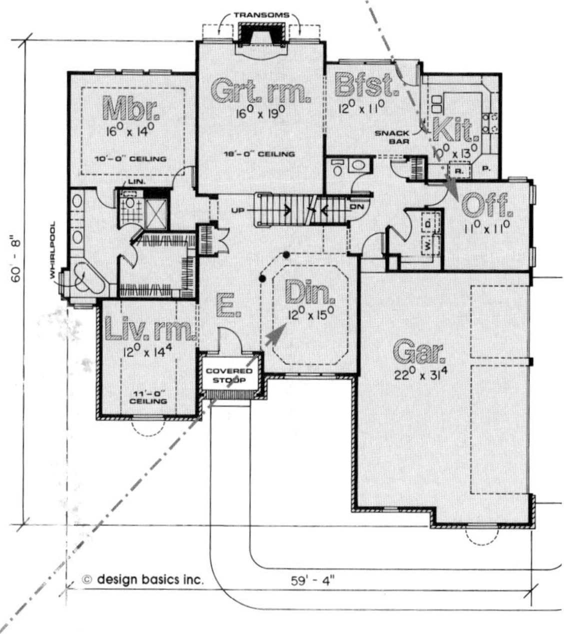

The open dining room blends with the entry, creating sense of openness.

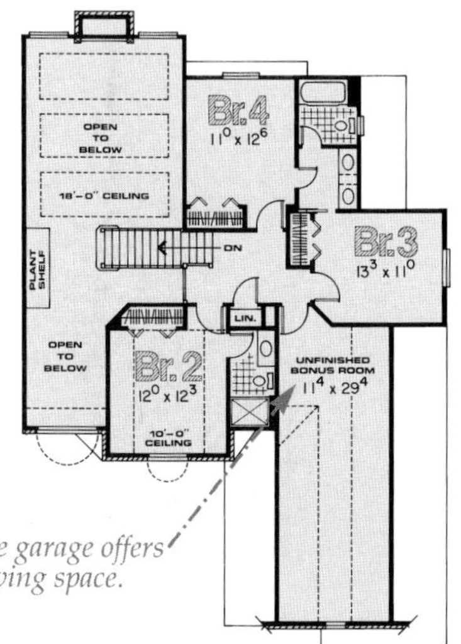

A bonus room above the garage offers additional storage or living space.

Bonus Room Adds 361 Square Feet

SCENIC OVERLOOK

Main Floor: 1519 Sq. Ft.
Second Floor: 594 Sq. Ft.
Total Square Feet: 2113 Sq. Ft.

Meredith

#28A-2312 Plan Price $545

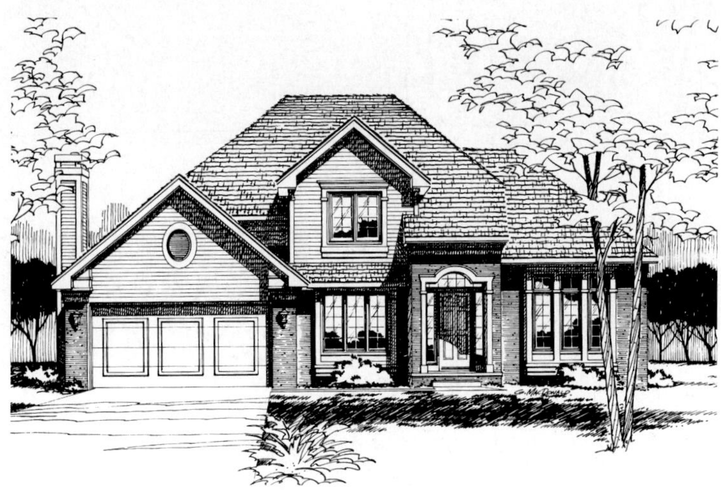

The kitchen, breakfast area and family room are well integrated for day-to-day living.

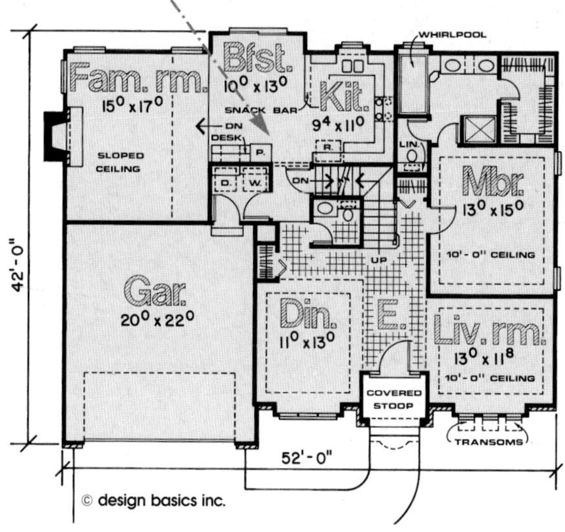

A loft overlooking the family room easily converts into a home office.

The potential for a bonus room above the garage leaves options for a fourth bedroom or exercise area.

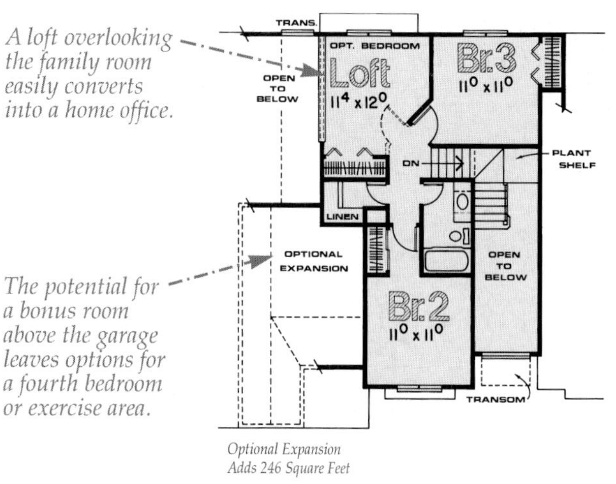

Optional Expansion Adds 246 Square Feet

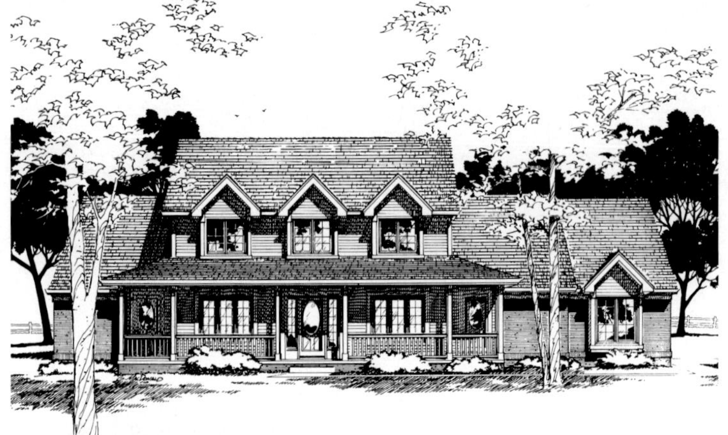

Easy options

Main Floor:	1881 Sq. Ft.
Second Floor:	814 Sq. Ft.
Total Square Feet:	2695 Sq. Ft.

Bridgeport

#28A-2460 Plan Price $595

With its built-in bookshelves, the living room easily converts into a den or office.

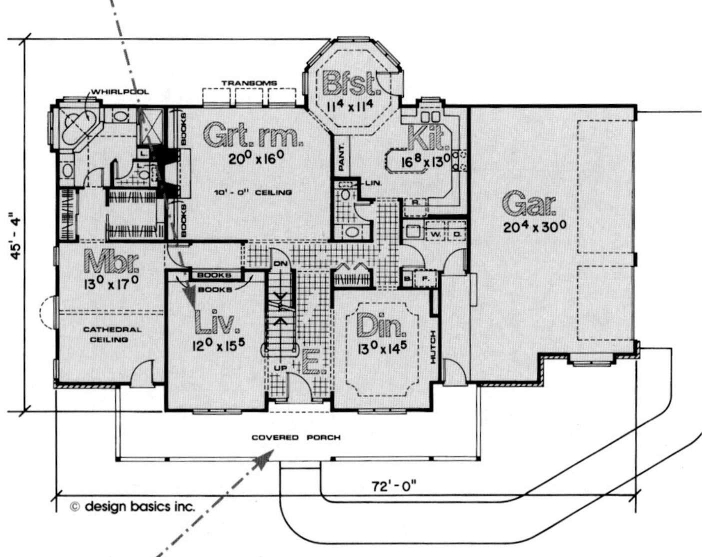

Spanning the front of the home, a deep porch has access from the master suite and garage.

A display gallery on the second floor is highlighted in the two-story entry with boxed ceiling.

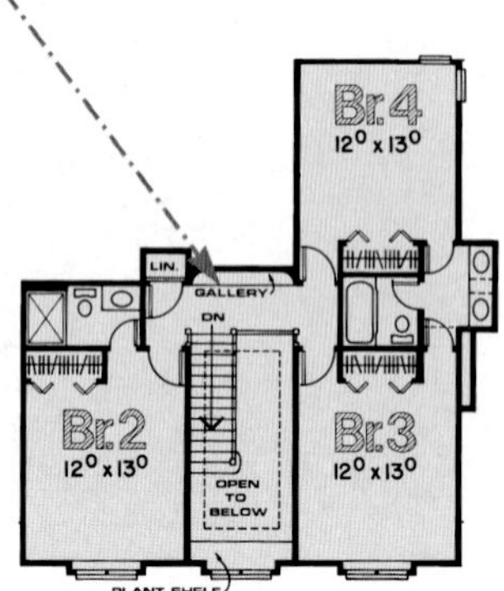

Dramatic den

Main Floor:	2555 Sq. Ft.
Second Floor:	1001 Sq. Ft.
Total Square Feet:	3556 Sq. Ft.

Winchester

#28A-2475 Plan Price $685

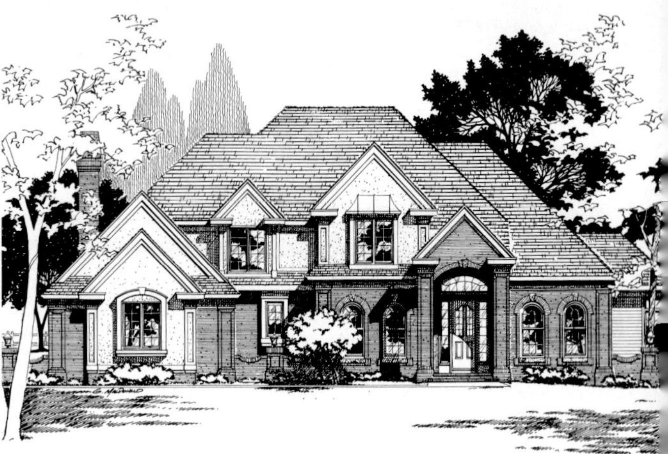

A sensible snack bar in the kitchen serves both the breakfast area and gathering room.

A skylight brightens the master suite's whirlpool tub. His and her walk-in closets are also featured.

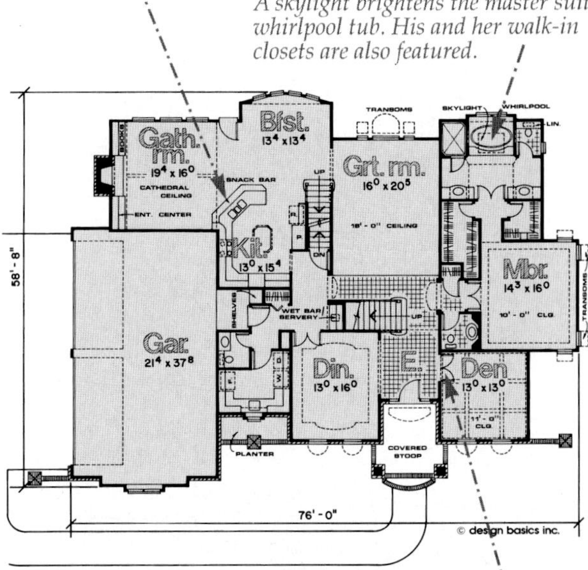

Double doors reveal the den with an 11-foot-high, spider-beamed ceiling

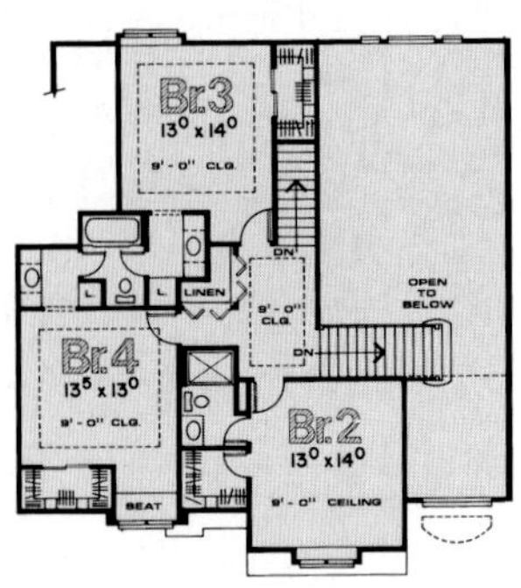

design basics inc. HOME PLAN DESIGN SERVICE

CONVERTIBLE BEDROOM

Lansing

Main Floor: 1517 Sq. Ft.
Second Floor: 431 Sq. Ft.
Total Square Feet: 1948 Sq. Ft.

#28A-2554 Plan Price $525

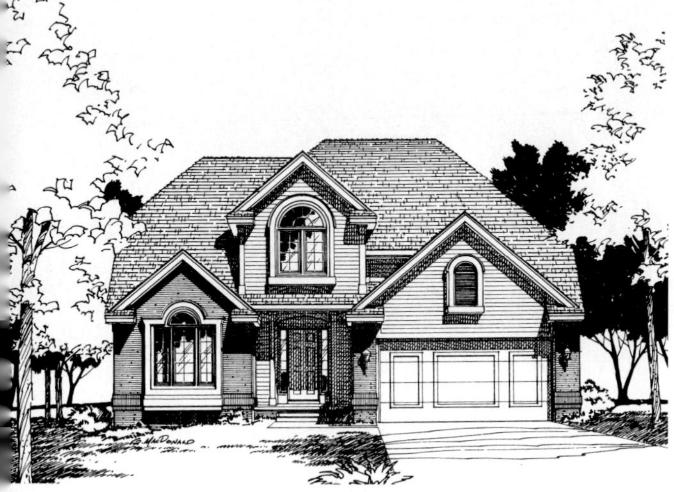

0-foot great
features a
fireplace
ll windows
back.

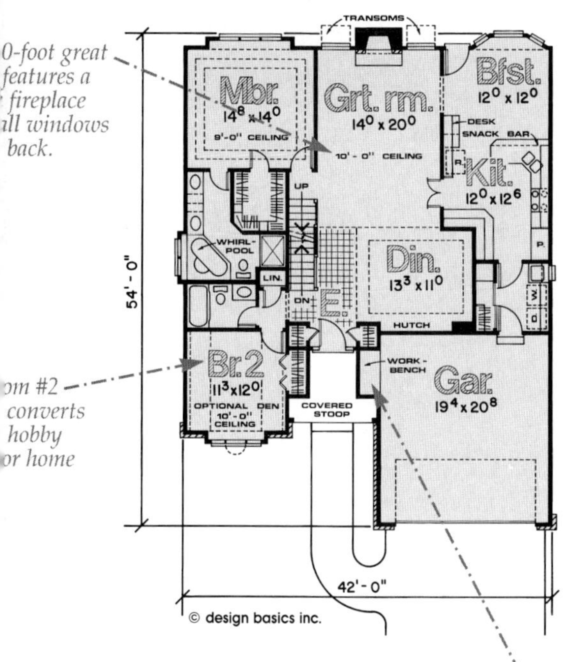

om #2
converts
hobby
or home

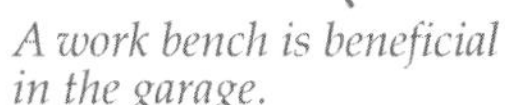

A work bench is beneficial in the garage.

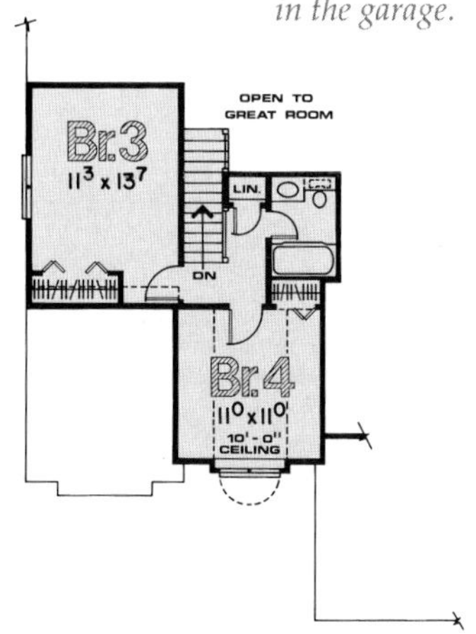

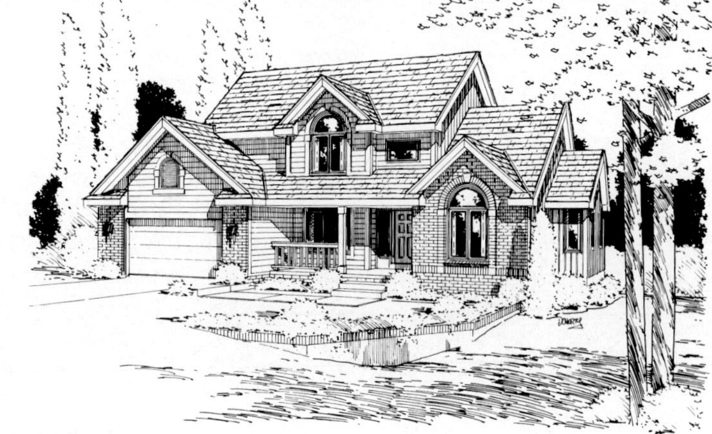

WELCOME WORK AREA

Crescent Creek

Main Floor: 1854 Sq. Ft.
Second Floor: 716 Sq. Ft.
Total Square Feet: 2570 Sq. Ft.

#28A-8127 Plan Price $485

The open kitchen, breakfast area and family room welcome today's casual living.

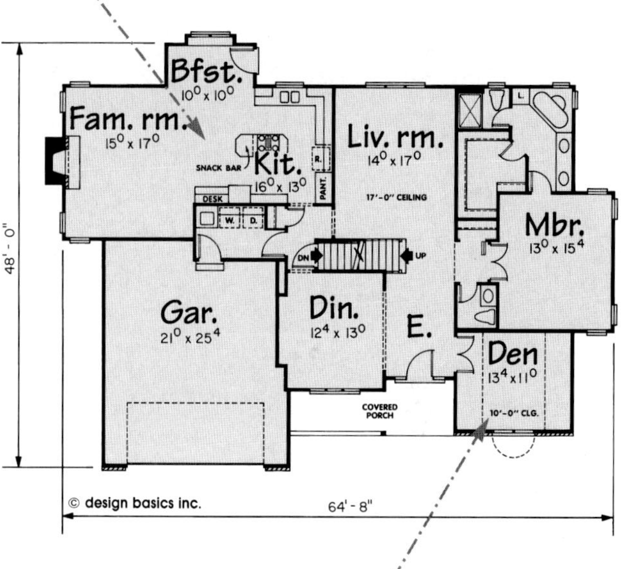

A volume ceiling and arched window enhance the den as a home office or second main-floor bedroom.

A compartmented bath serves three roomy second floor bedrooms.

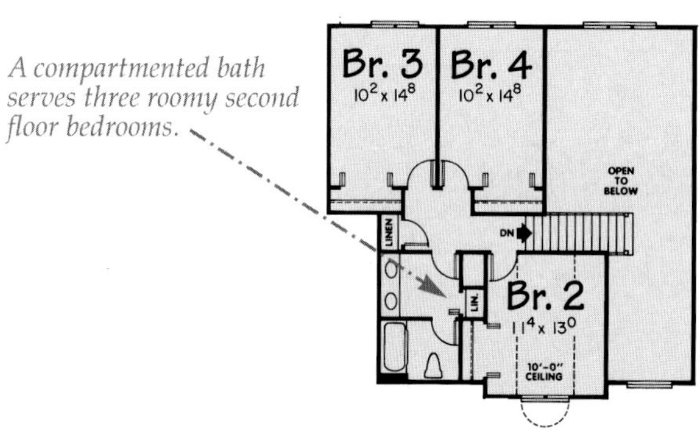

Room For Storage . . . *Ask most of us what we would like to change about our current home and we'd most likely say, 'There's not enough room for storage.' One can never have enough, it seems – especially when many of the things we've accumulated are too valuable to get rid of. The following plans feature a variety of storage.*

Imagination Space

Main Floor: 1597 Sq. Ft.
Second Floor: 685 Sq. Ft.
Total Square Feet: 2282 Sq. Ft.

Tanner

#28A-3249 Plan Price $555

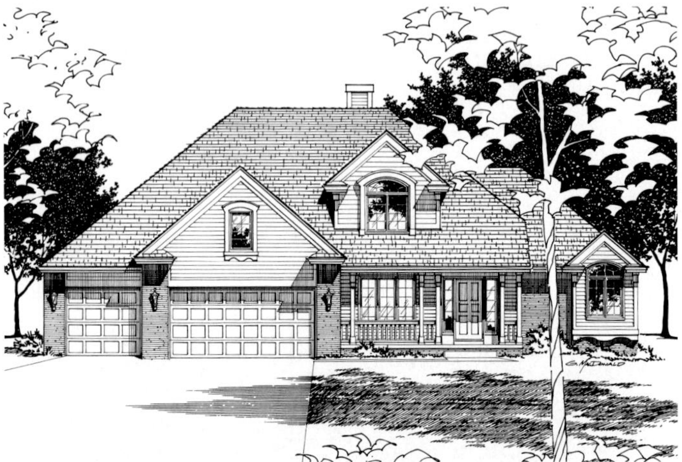

A see-thru fireplace adds warmth to the great room and breakfast area.

A window seat adds romance to the master bath.

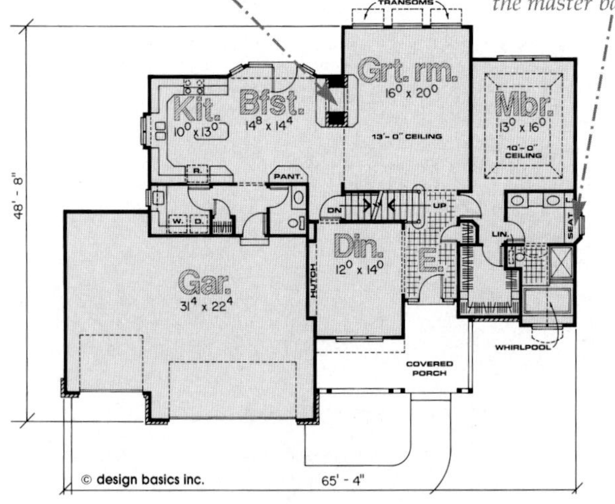

A window brightens the second floor bonus room, adding more than 300 square feet of living space.

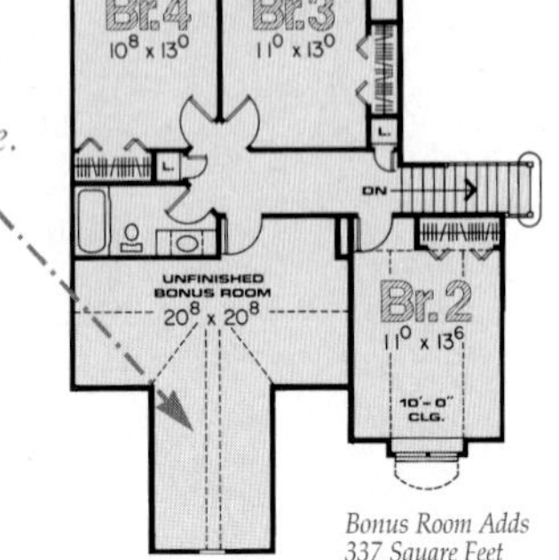

Bonus Room Adds 337 Square Feet

design basics inc. HOME PLAN DESIGN SERVICE

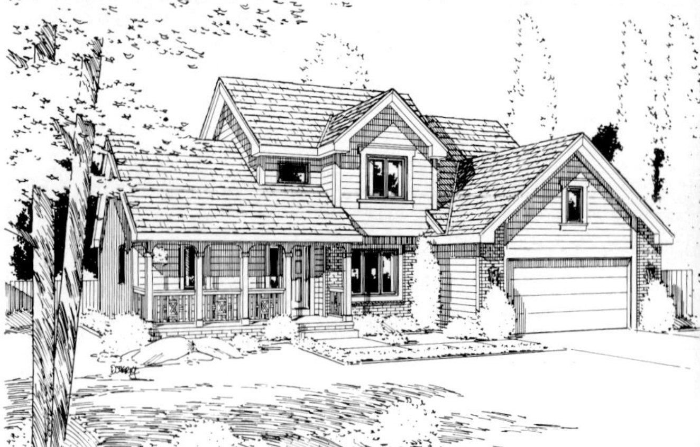

A Place for Your "Stuff"

Main Floor: 1301 Sq. Ft.
Second Floor: 564 Sq. Ft.
Total Square Feet: 1865 Sq. Ft.

Brook Valley

#28A-8084 Plan Price $415

The well-connected kitchen, dinette, and great room are perfect for today's practical living.

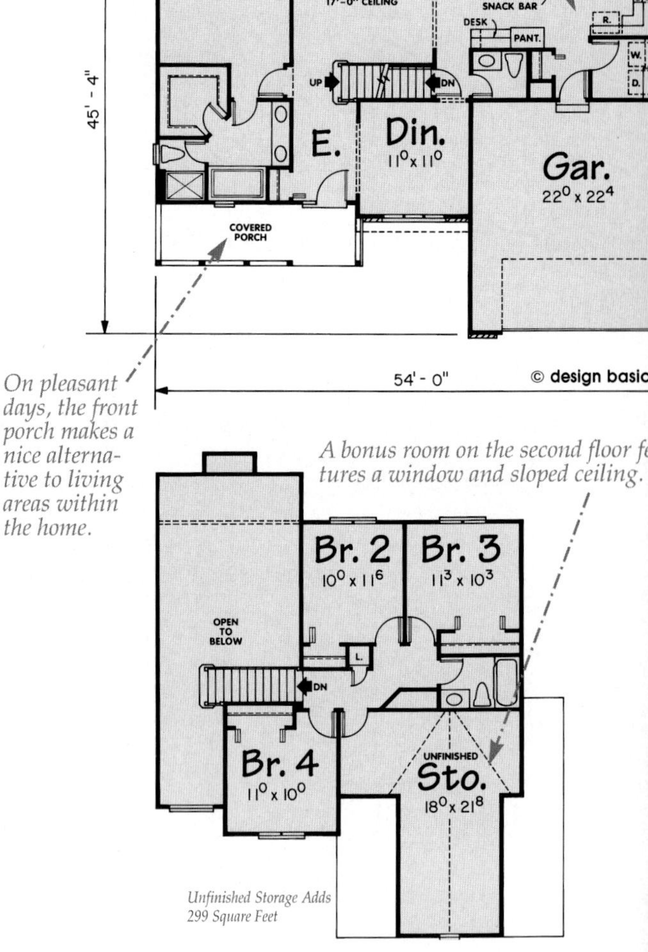

On pleasant days, the front porch makes a nice alternative to living areas within the home.

A bonus room on the second floor features a window and sloped ceiling.

Unfinished Storage Adds 299 Square Feet

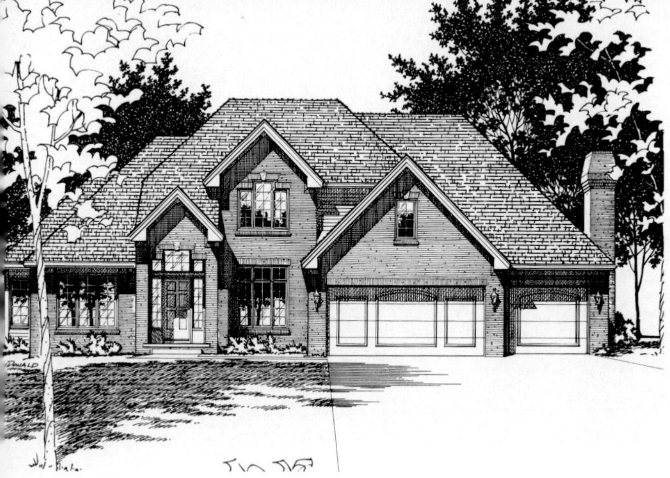

GENEROUS BONUS ROOM

Main Floor: 2179 Sq. Ft.
Second Floor: 838 Sq. Ft.
Total Square Feet: 3017 Sq. Ft.

Oakdale

#28A-3326 Plan Price $635

spectacular window creates
we in the living room.

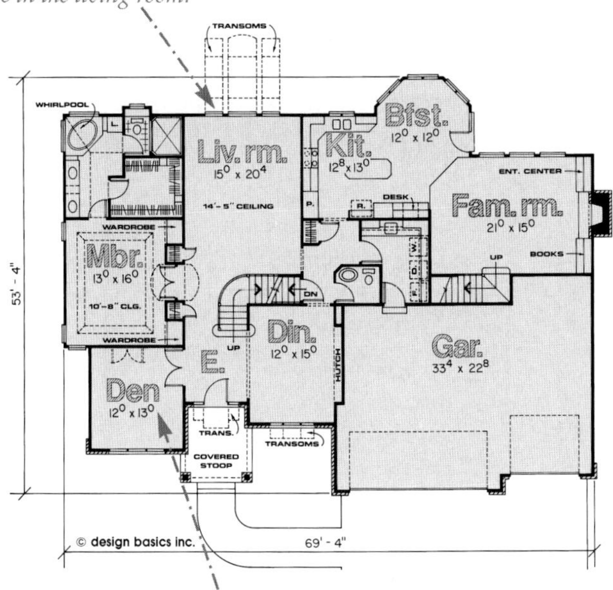

Perfect for the home office, the den is also accessible to the master bedroom through French doors.

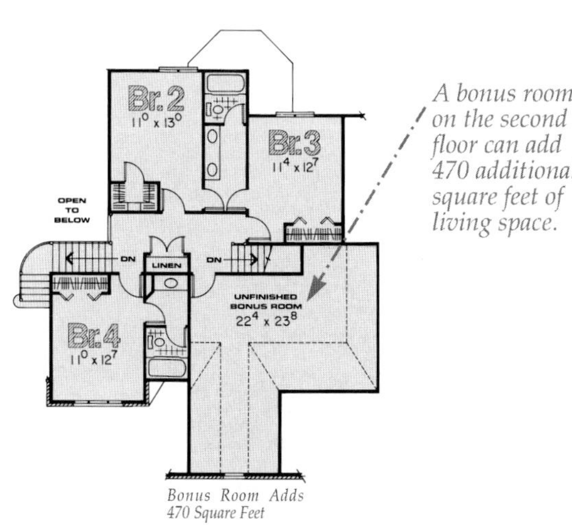

A bonus room on the second floor can add 470 additional square feet of living space.

Bonus Room Adds
470 Square Feet

STORAGE UP AND DOWN

Main Floor: 1348 Sq. Ft.
Second Floor: 609 Sq. Ft.
Total Square Feet: 1957 Sq. Ft.

Taylor

#28A-3063 Plan Price $525

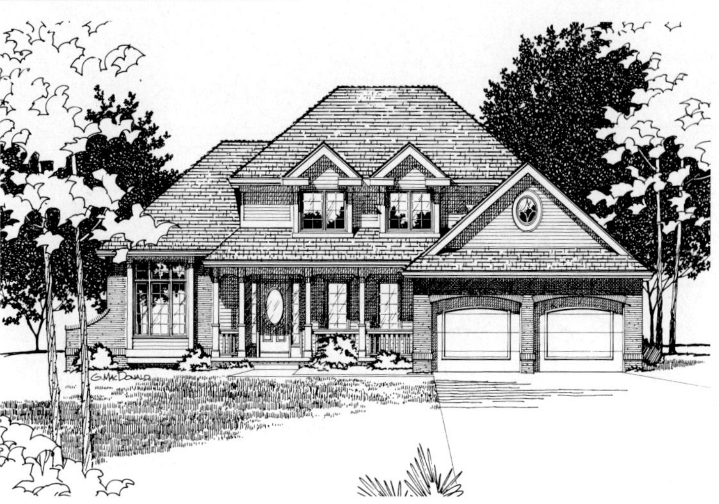

Tall windows on either side of the fireplace offer a welcoming atmosphere in the family room.

Storage space in the garage leaves room for bikes, lawn mowers and other equipment.

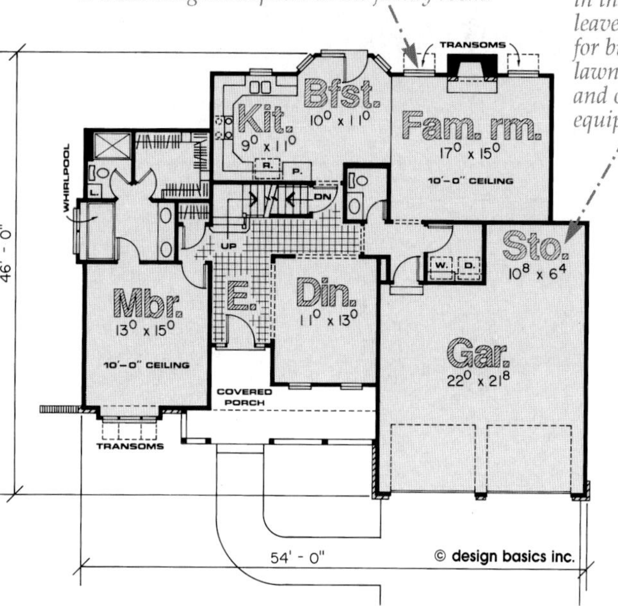

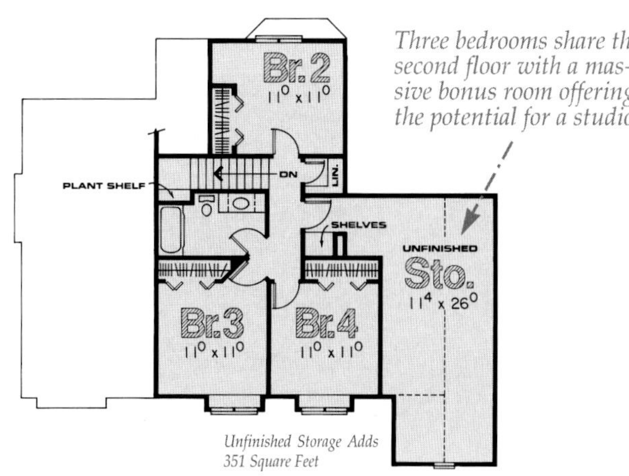

Three bedrooms share the second floor with a massive bonus room offering the potential for a studio.

Unfinished Storage Adds
351 Square Feet

*A*N EXPANSE FOR EXPANSION

Main Floor: 1878 Sq. Ft.
Second Floor: 719 Sq. Ft.
Total Square Feet: 2597 Sq. Ft.

Addams

#28A-3510 Plan Price $585

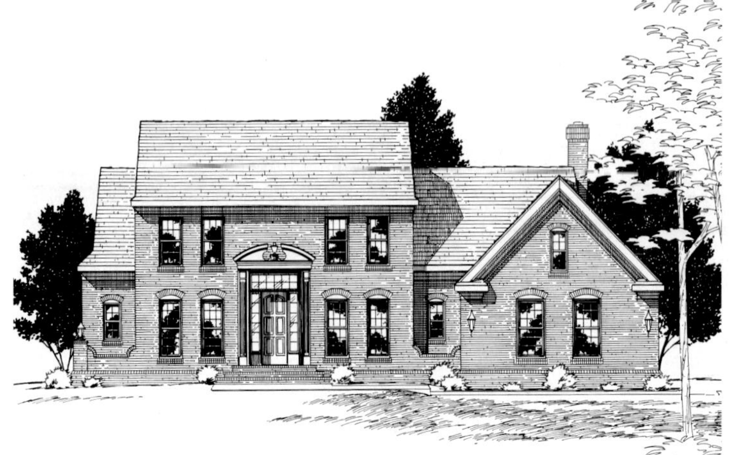

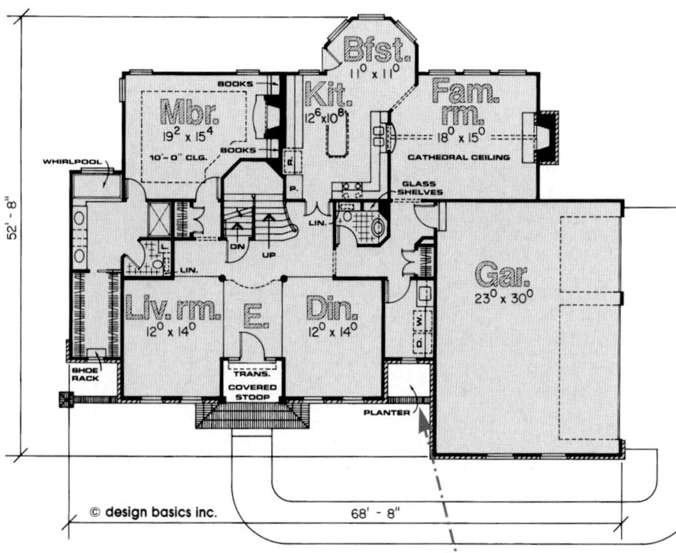

A balcony enjoys a view of the two-story entry.

A decorative planter beautifies the front elevation.

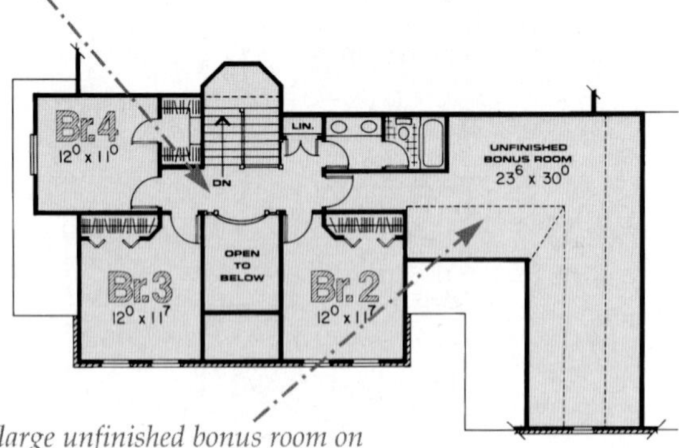

A large unfinished bonus room on the second floor provides an area for storage or possible expansion.

Unfinished Storage Adds 542 Square Feet

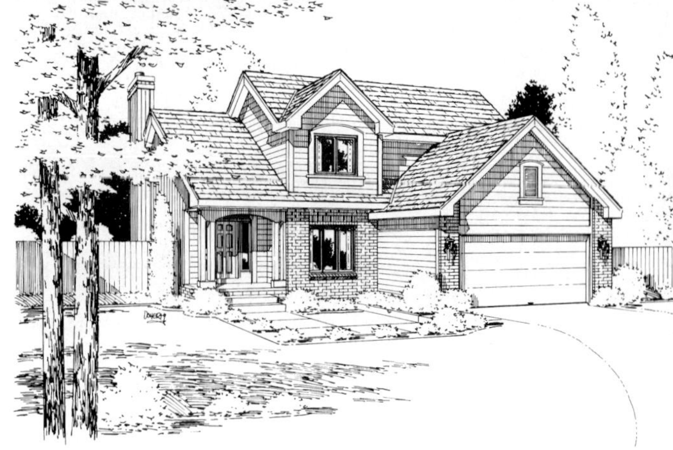

*S*EASONAL HIDEAWAY

Main Floor: 1324 Sq. Ft.
Second Floor: 391 Sq. Ft.
Total Square Feet: 1715 Sq. Ft.

Angel Cove

#28A-8094 Plan Price $405

Bayed windows in the breakfast area provide a perfect view of the outdoors from the kitchen.

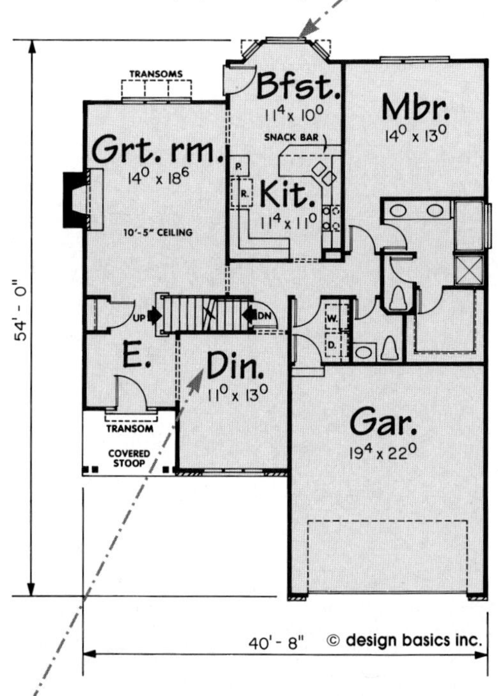

The dining room is within steps of the kitchen for convenience.

A bonus room on the second floor offers plenty of storage for seasonal and other items

Unfinished Bonus Room Adds 212 Square Feet

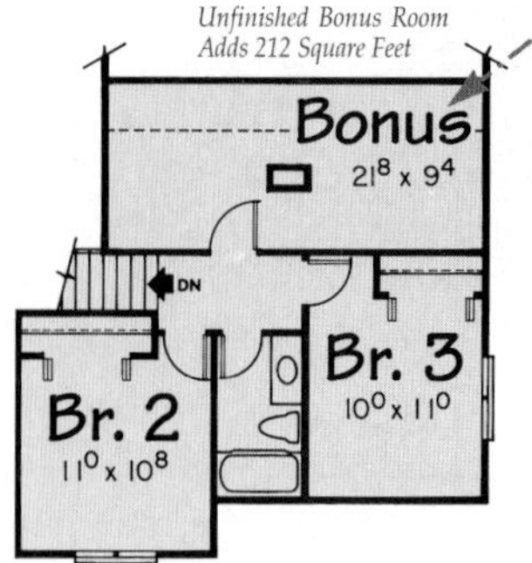

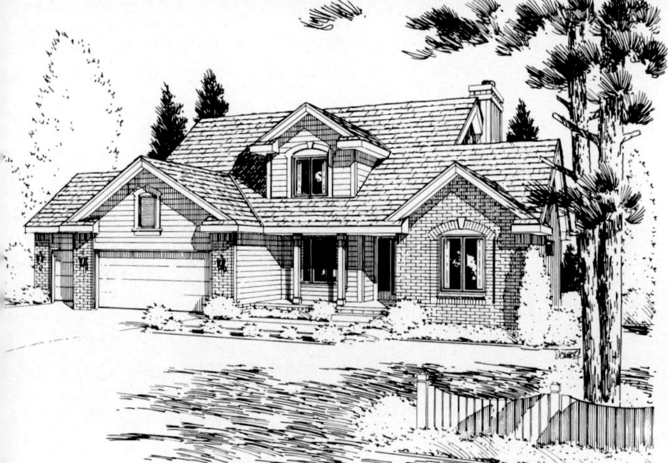

ROOM TO GROW

Main Floor: 1411 Sq. Ft.
Second Floor: 618 Sq. Ft.
Total Square Feet: 2029 Sq. Ft.

Hannifan Lane

#28A-8065 Plan Price $435

Well integrated with the kitchen and breakfast area, the great room features a tall transom window and fireplace.

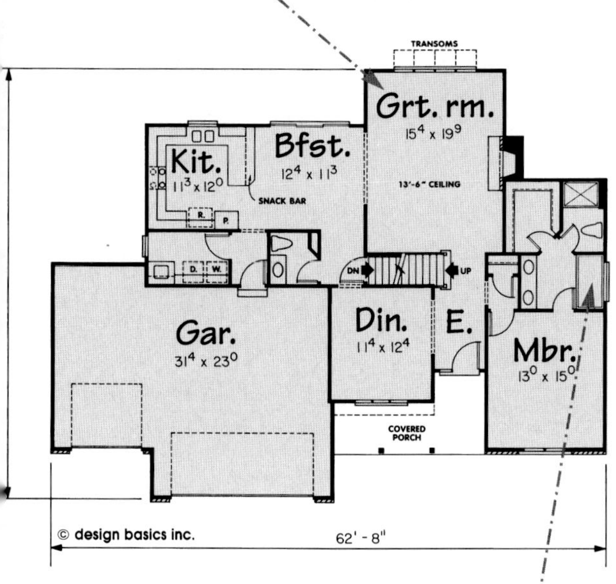

A soaking tub across from a dual-lav vanity accompanies a relaxing master suite.

A large bonus room provides extra storage or living space on the second floor.

Br. 3
10^9 x 11^3
Br. 4
10^9 x 11^3
OPEN TO BELOW
L
DN
Bonus
20^4 x 10^0
Br. 2
11^4 x 11^4

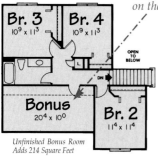

Unfinished Bonus Room Adds 214 Square Feet

HOME IMPROVEMENT SPACE

Main Floor: 1653 Sq. Ft.
Second Floor: 700 Sq. Ft.
Total Square Feet: 2353 Sq. Ft.

Manchester

#28A-1862 Plan Price $565

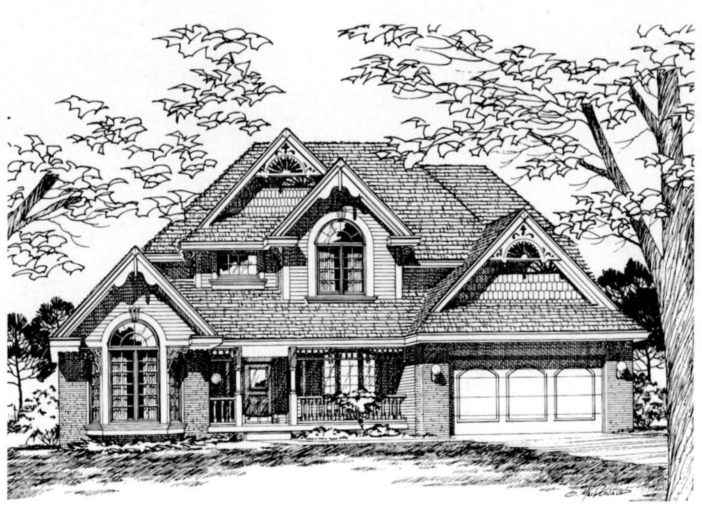

A see-thru fireplace and bookshelf create a relaxing atmosphere in the hearth room/kitchen.

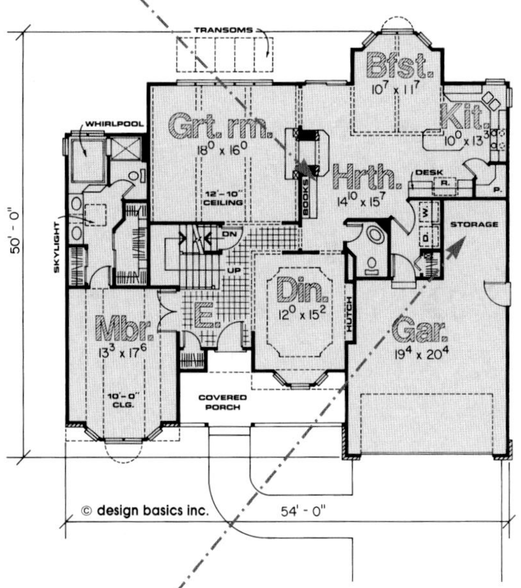

A large storage area in the garage leaves room for a workbench and home improvement projects.

A walk-in closet in bedroom #2 offers the potential for additional seasonal storage.

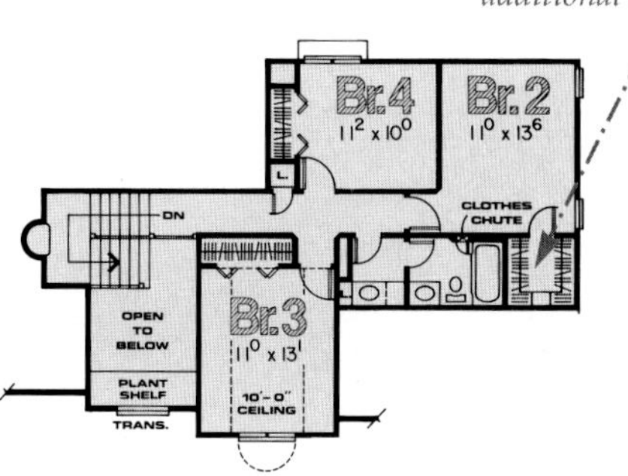

An avid collector of antiques, I cherish my mother's three-piece Eastlake settee and early 1800s storage bench in ways that perhaps most would not. Most people probably take their heritage for granted, having grown up with family reunions and visiting grandparents. I never knew these things as a child. My family moved around a lot (I attended many different schools), rarely settling in one place for more than a couple of years. My father was self-employed, forcing us to move on as his business would decline. I did not grow up knowing my aunts, uncles and cousins. I barely knew my grandparents. And it's because of this, that my memories and heritage are so important to me now.

My family moved around a lot (I attended many different schools), rarely settling in one place for more than a couple of years. My father was self-employed forcing us to move on as his business would decline.

My life holds its meaning in these memories, in the roots of my family. And they are

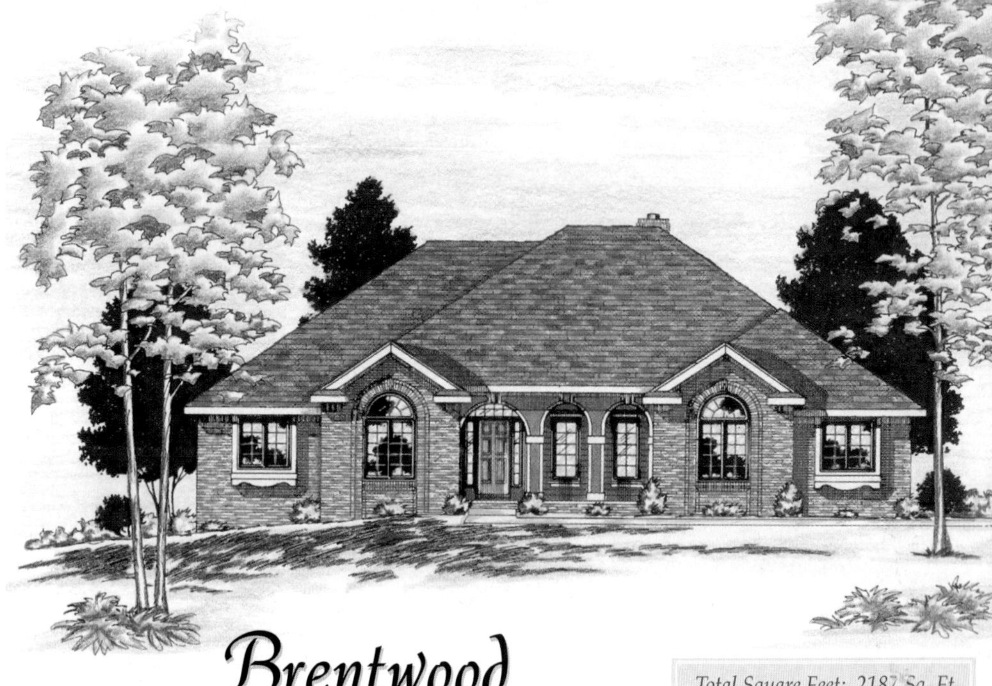

Brentwood

Total Square Feet: 2187 Sq. Ft.

#28A-3598 Plan Price $545

The great room is designed for entertaining with its see-thru fireplace, large windows, entertainment center and convenient access to the wet bar.

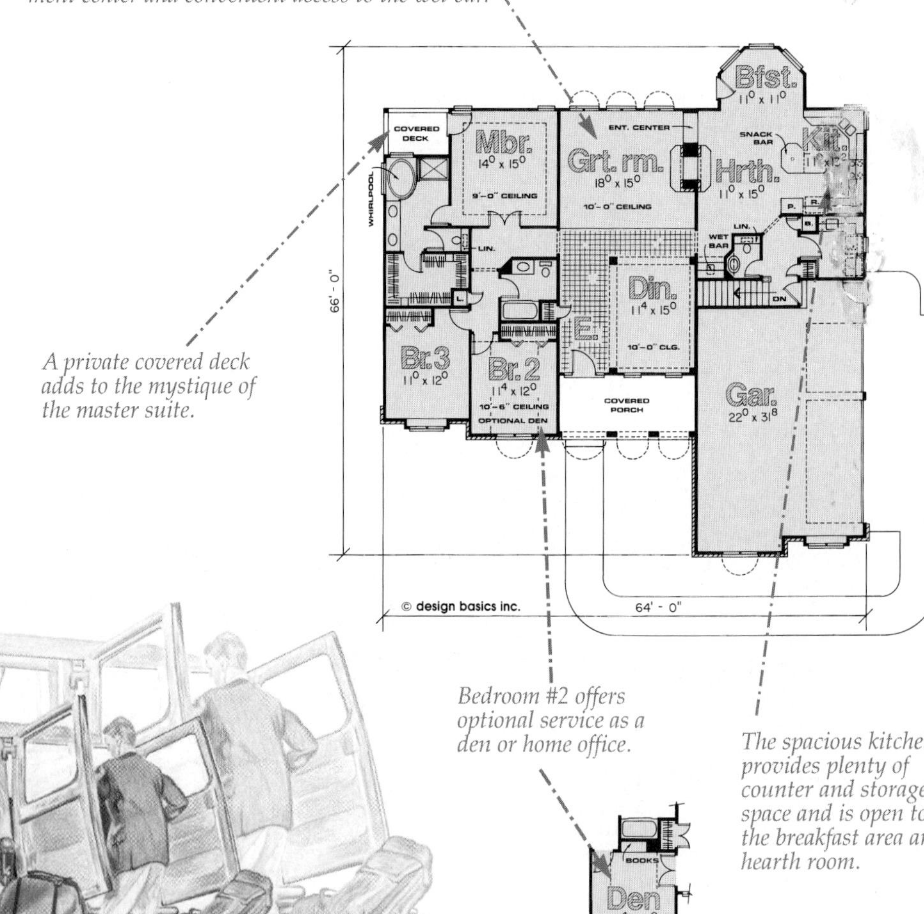

A private covered deck adds to the mystique of the master suite.

Bedroom #2 offers optional service as a den or home office.

The spacious kitchen provides plenty of counter and storage space and is open to the breakfast area an hearth room.

design basics inc. HOME PLAN DESIGN SERVICE

dear to me for reasons much more compelling, now that I'm older and our youngest son is ready to leave home. I cling to them as tightly as I will hold my son before he walks out the door to find his first job, a lasting love, and his place in the scheme of life. And with his leaving, we anticipate building a new home – a new place to house my roots.

The walls of my current home are alive with memories. They are decorated with old photographs and keepsakes from my relatives' past. One of my favorites is a collage I created for my husband with memorabilia from his family – a camera lens from his uncle, a photography buff; a Purple Heart Medal from his father, a veteran of WWII; a baby shoe from his aunt; his grandfather's Bible and a Valentine's day card from his father to his mother during the war. I have likewise created collages of my own family, my grandmothers and long-gone cherished friends. For me, these living essays are a recourse for the many years I spent ungrounded. They help remind me of where I've been, and who was there before me.

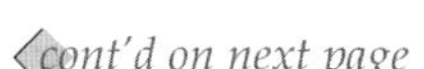

cont'd on next page

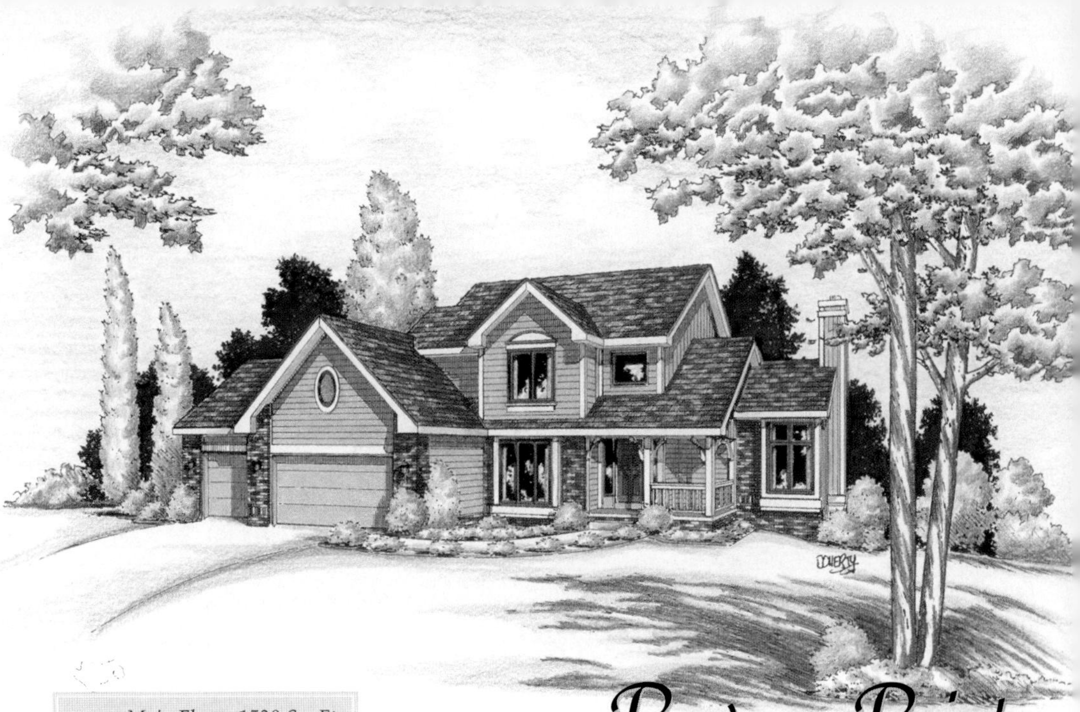

Pawnee Point

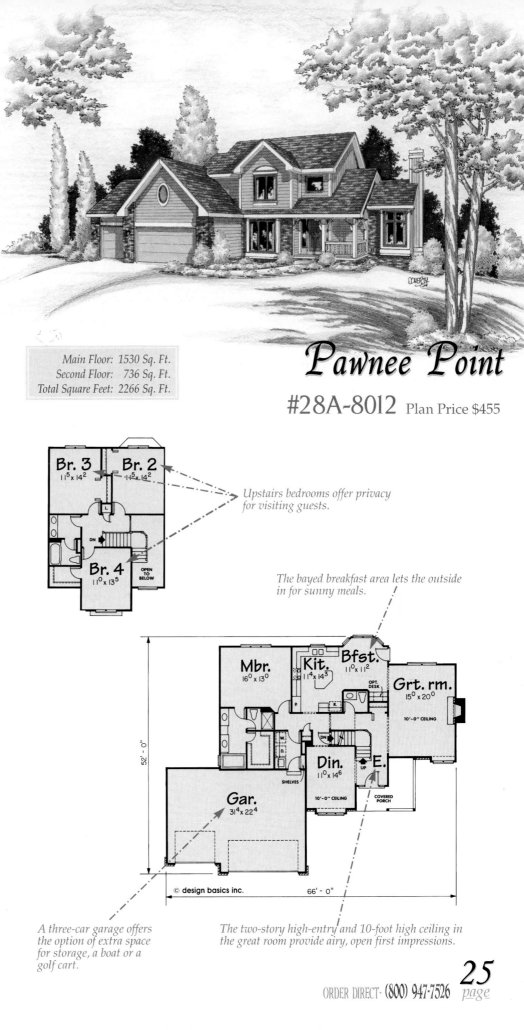

Main Floor:	1530 Sq. Ft.
Second Floor:	736 Sq. Ft.
Total Square Feet:	2266 Sq. Ft.

#28A-8012 Plan Price $455

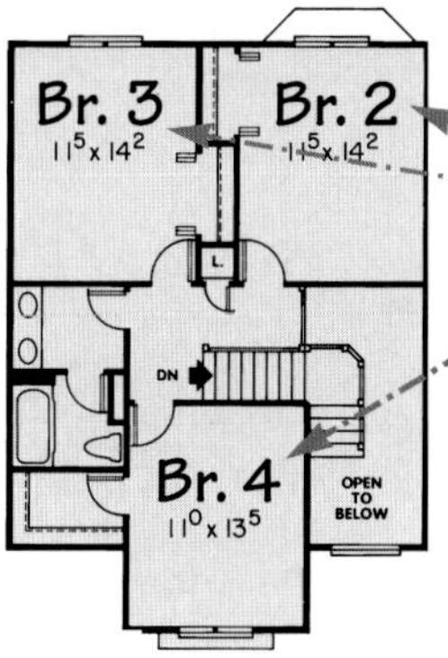

Br. 3 11⁵ x 14²
Br. 2 11⁵ x 14²
Br. 4 11⁰ x 13⁵
DN
OPEN TO BELOW

Upstairs bedrooms offer privacy for visiting guests.

The bayed breakfast area lets the outside in for sunny meals.

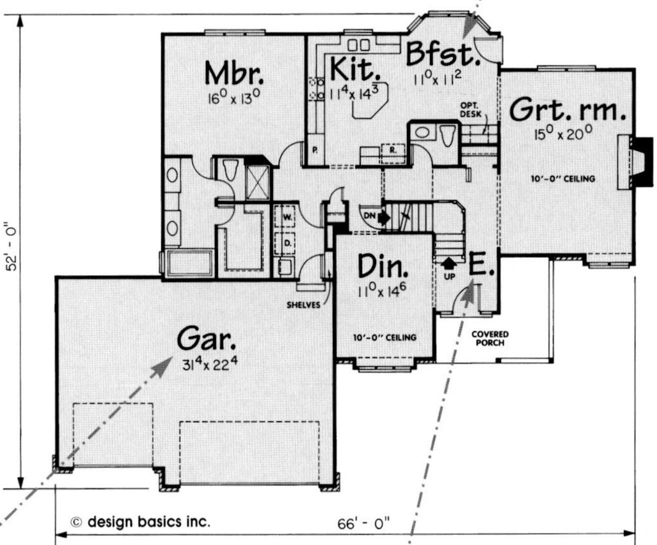

Mbr. 16⁰ x 13⁰
Kit. 11⁴ x 14³
Bfst. 11⁰ x 11²
OPT. DESK
Grt. rm. 15⁰ x 20⁰
10'-0" CEILING
W. D.
DN
Din. 11⁰ x 14⁶
10'-0" CEILING
UP
E.
SHELVES
COVERED PORCH
Gar. 31⁴ x 22⁴
52' - 0"
66' - 0"

© design basics inc.

A three-car garage offers the option of extra space for storage, a boat or a golf cart.

The two-story high-entry and 10-foot high ceiling in the great room provide airy, open first impressions.

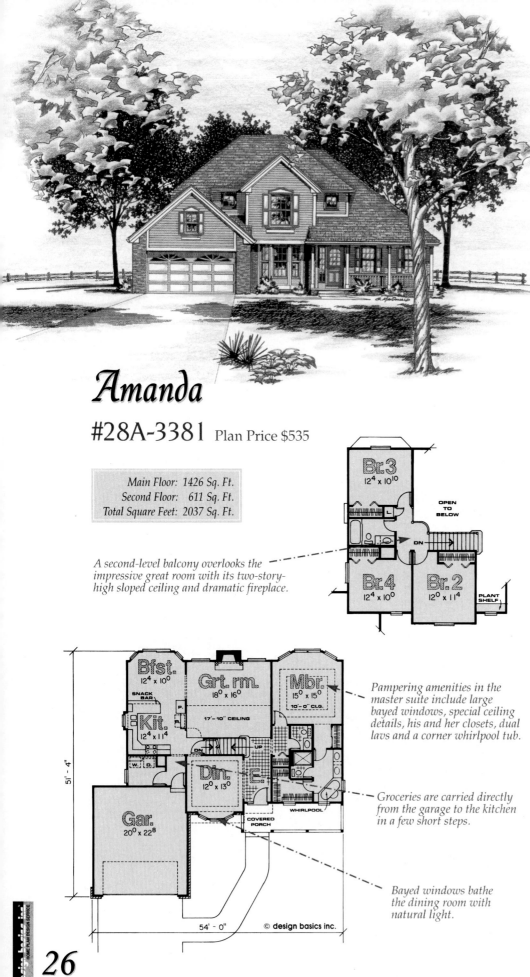

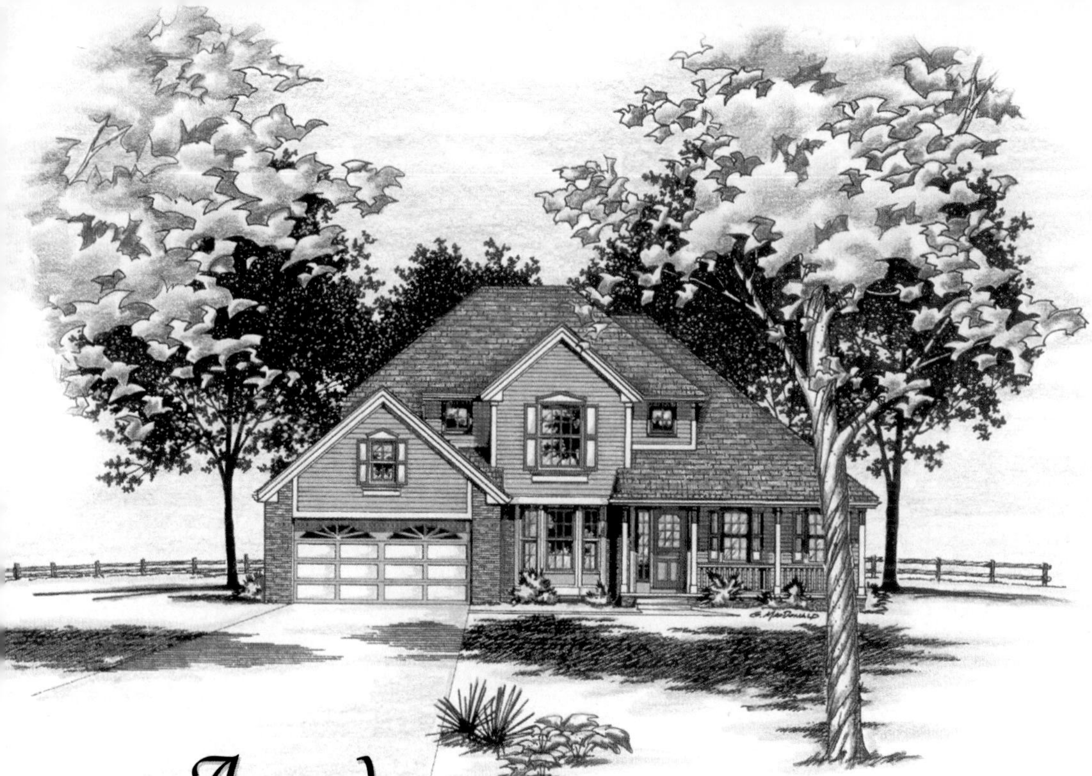

Amanda

#28A-3381 Plan Price $535

Main Floor:	1426 Sq. Ft.
Second Floor:	611 Sq. Ft.
Total Square Feet:	2037 Sq. Ft.

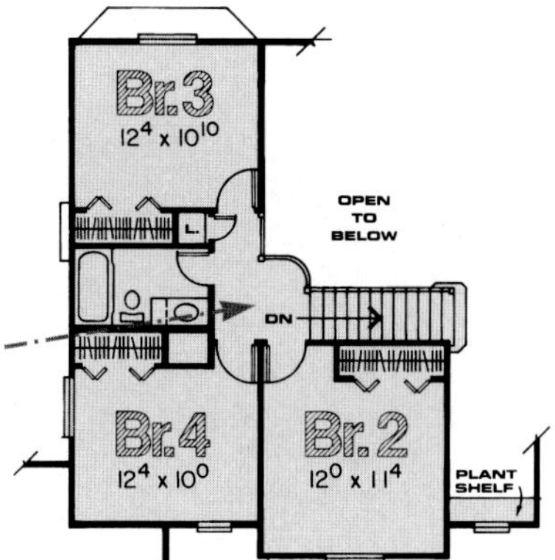

A second-level balcony overlooks the impressive great room with its two-story-high sloped ceiling and dramatic fireplace.

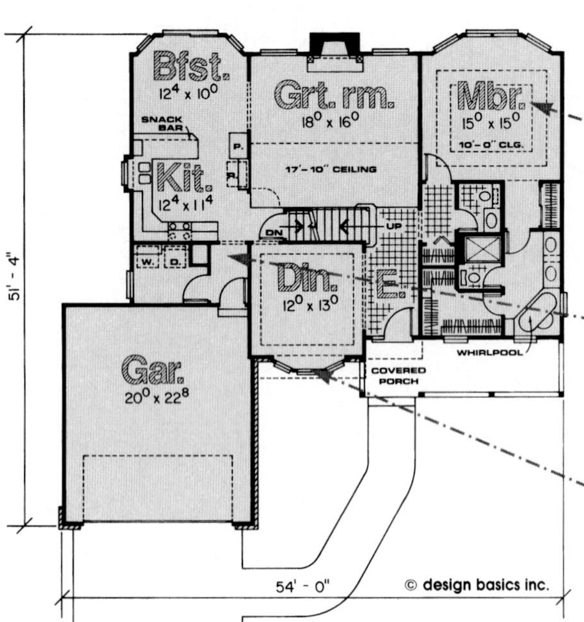

Pampering amenities in the master suite include large bayed windows, special ceiling details, his and her closets, dual lavs and a corner whirlpool tub.

Groceries are carried directly from the garage to the kitchen in a few short steps.

Bayed windows bathe the dining room with natural light.

© design basics inc.

The walls of my current home are alive with memories. They are decorated with old photographs and keepsakes from my relatives' past.

They are symbols of my legacy, creating the foundation upon which I stand. I came to realize years later that it was an inner strength drawn from this foundation that urged me to finally get my college degree just a few years ago. It prompted me to own an aerobics' studio. It directed me to leave the comfort of a job I held for 14 years, and move into the unknown territory of a fledgling company. These symbols will follow me into my new home and lay the foundation for our future.

I do not yet know what our new home will look like, but I know it must be large. I live in a central location between my mother, brother and sister, so my house

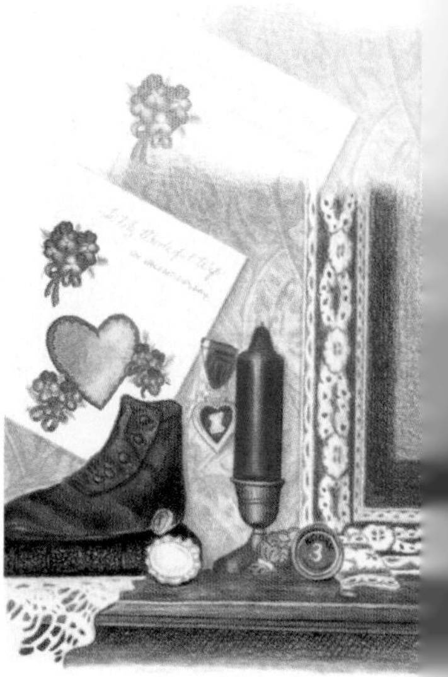

cont'd on next page

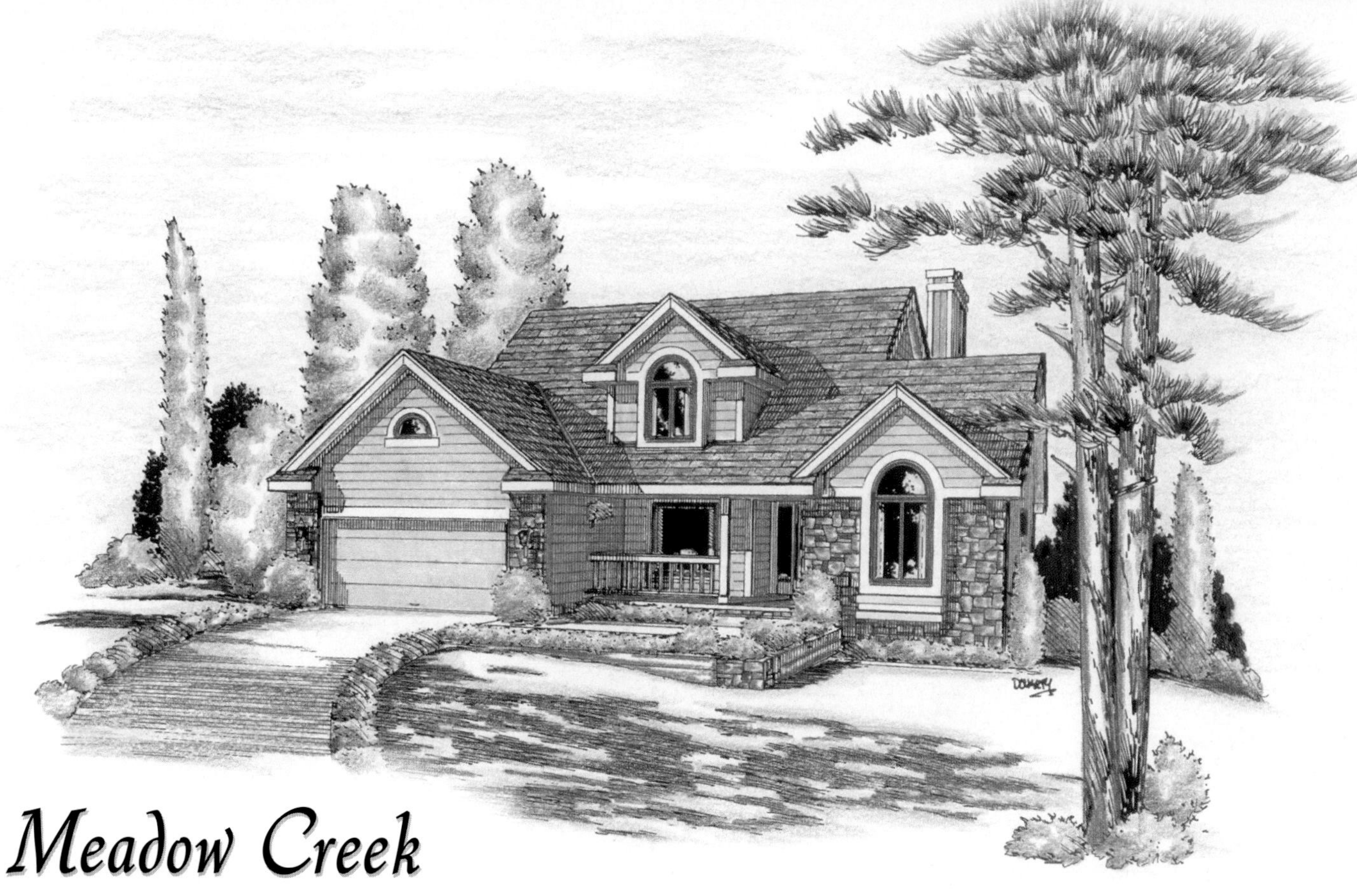

Meadow Creek

#28A-8077 Plan Price $415

Secondary bedrooms are situated upstairs and opposite the main-floor master suite to ensure privacy.

Views from the kitchen/breakfast area center on the great room's fireplace.

TRANSOMS

Grt. rm. 15^{4} x 19^{8}

13'-0" CEILING

Kit. 13^{4} x 11^{3}

SNACK BAR

Bfst. 11^{0} x 11^{3}

R. P. L. D. W.

DN UP

Din. 11^{4} x 11^{8}

E.

Mbr. 13^{0} x 16^{0}

10'-0" CLG.

Gar. 20^{8} x 23^{0}

COVERED PORCH

47' - 4"

52' - 0"

© design basics inc.

Br. 2 12^{7} x 11^{4}

OPEN TO GREAT ROOM

DN

L.

UNFINISHED Bonus 15^{0} x 23^{0}

Br. 3 11^{4} x 11^{4}

10'-0" CEILING

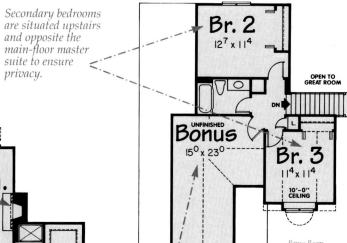

Bonus Room Adds 300 Sq. Ft.

An unfinished bonus room adds 300 square feet of space for a variety of needs.

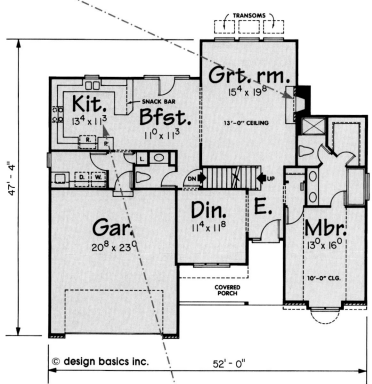

Main Floor: 1405 Sq. Ft.
Second Floor: 453 Sq. Ft.
Total Square Feet: 1858 Sq. Ft.

Direct access from garage to kitchen has a number of practical benefits.

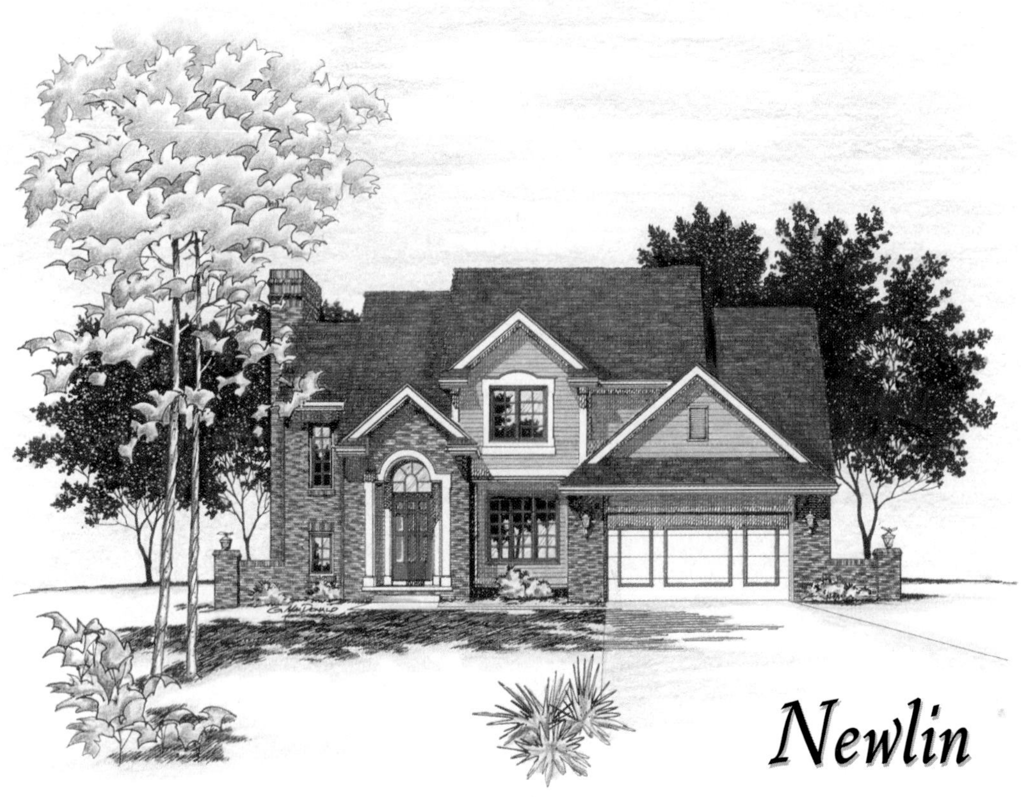

Newlin

#28A-2951 Plan Price $545

Main Floor:	1406 Sq. Ft.
Second Floor:	703 Sq. Ft.
Total Square Feet:	2109 Sq. Ft.

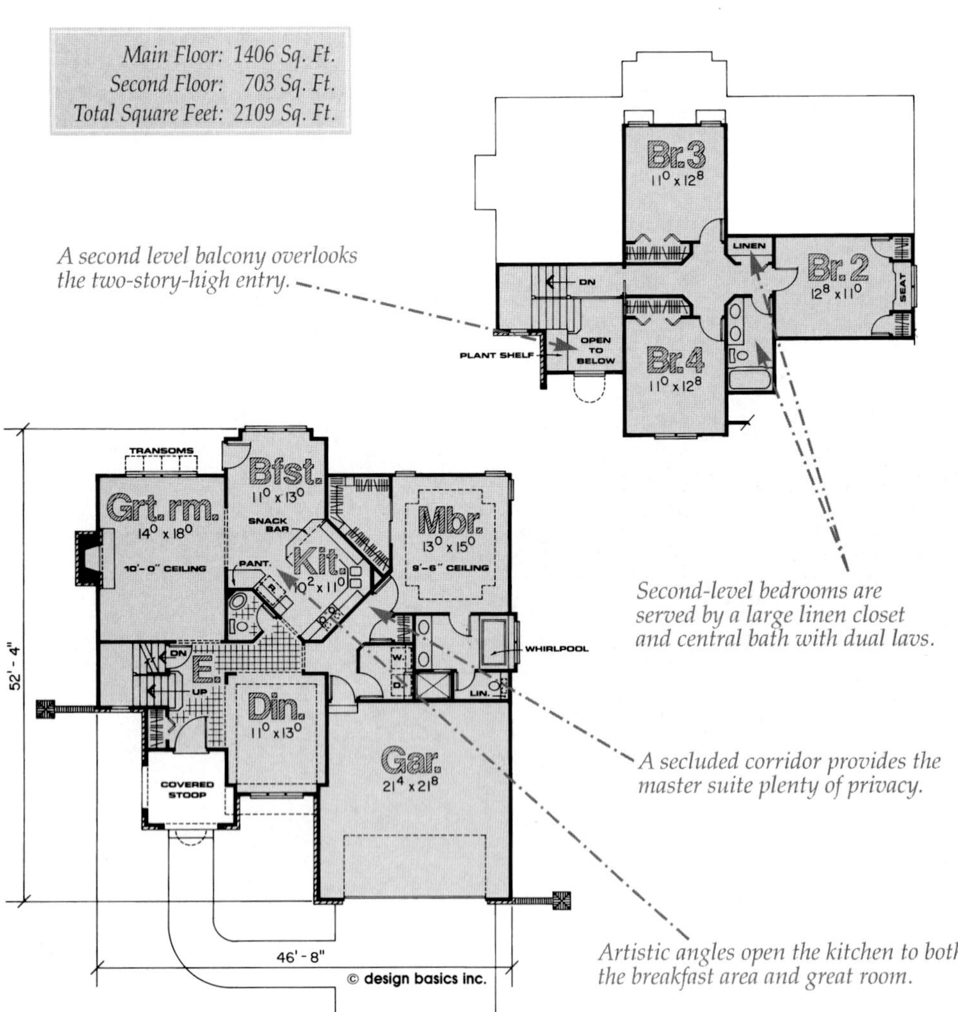

A second level balcony overlooks the two-story-high entry.

Second-level bedrooms are served by a large linen closet and central bath with dual lavs.

A secluded corridor provides the master suite plenty of privacy.

Artistic angles open the kitchen to both the breakfast area and great room.

I live in a central location between my mother, brother and sister, so my house is the place for our family get-togethers.

is the place for our family get-togethers. And besides accommodating my own children (and the friends and significant others they inevitably bring along), we frequently entertain friends, neighbors and business associates. My new home must be a place for them all.

My guests must be able to flow in and out of its rooms effortlessly. It must stimulate and accommodate. It must have just one bedroom on the main level and two formal areas for my antiques. It must have a kitchen that functions for a cook, yet acts like a living space. It must have guest rooms for my children and family to stay. It must not only

cont'd on next page

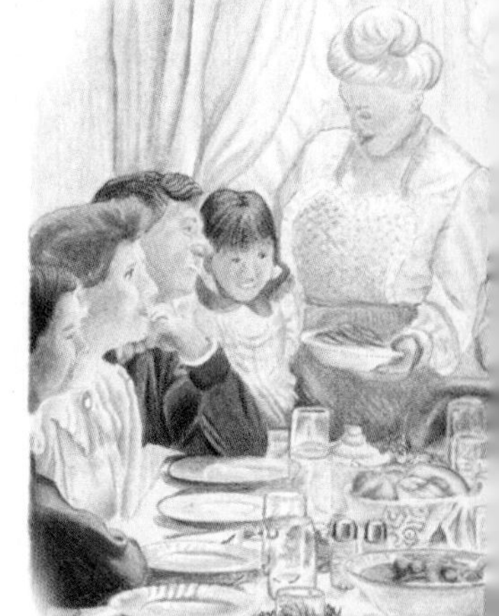

design basics inc. HOME PLAN DESIGN SERVICE

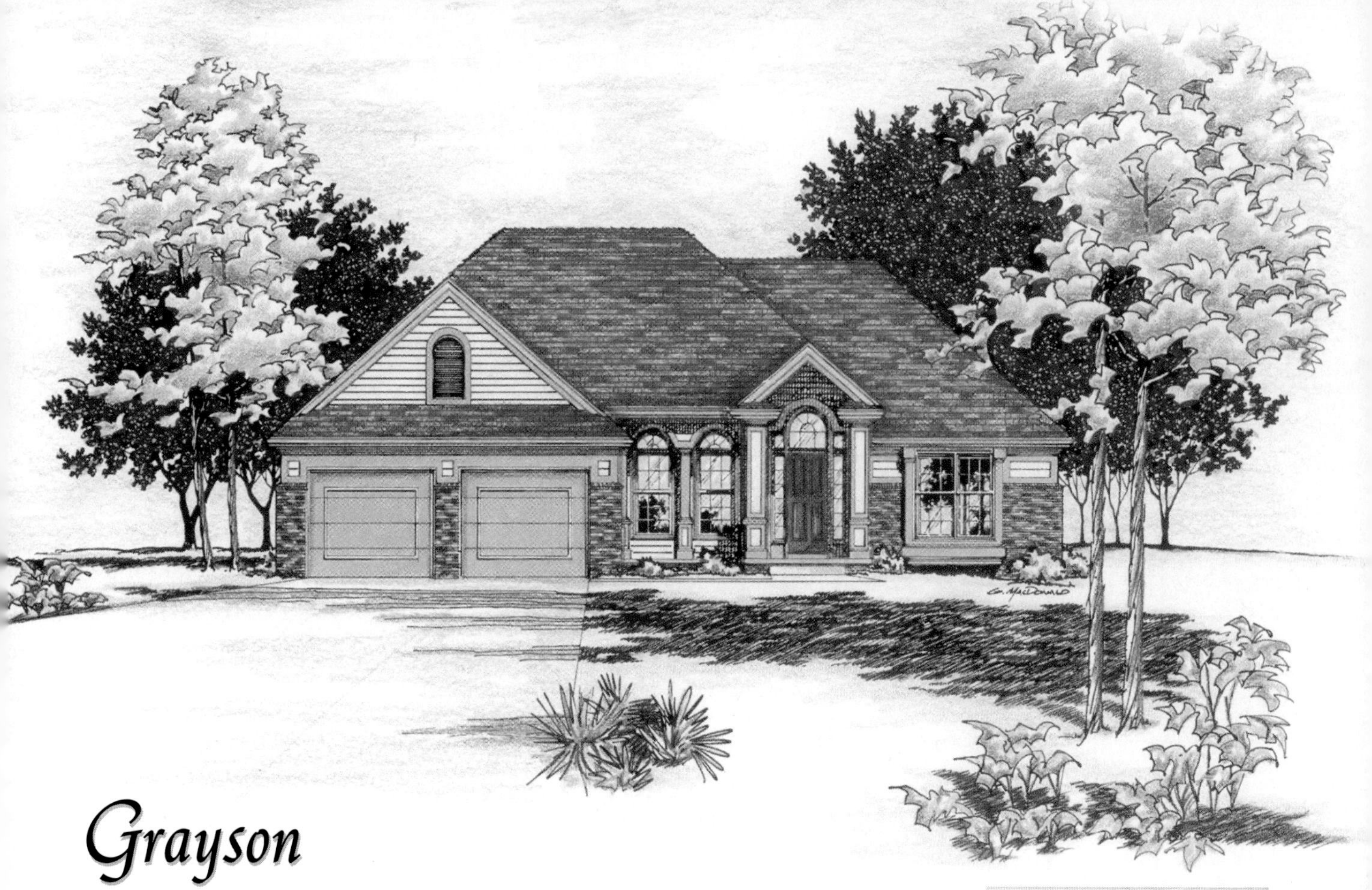

Grayson

#28A-3006 Plan Price $515

Total Square Feet: 1806 Sq. Ft.

The island kitchen boasts a pantry and plenty of counter space.

Built-in shelves provide added storage space in the garage.

The formal dining room is graced by a tiered ceiling and expansive views to the great room.

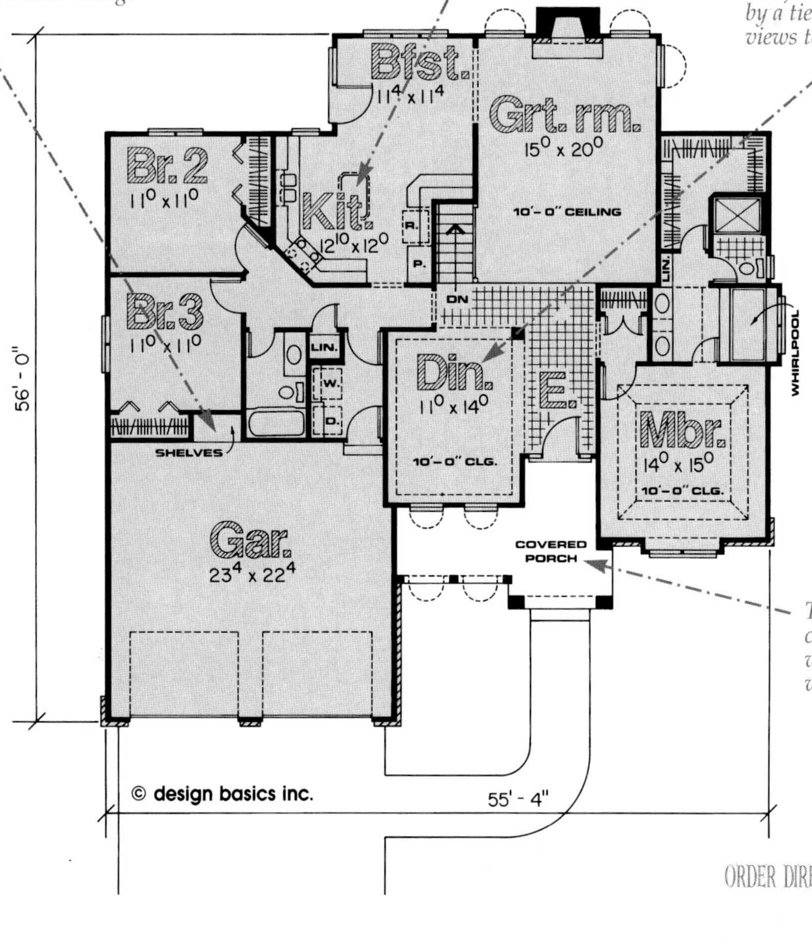

Bfst. $11^4 \times 11^4$

Grt. rm. $15^0 \times 20^0$

10'-0" CEILING

Br. 2 $11^0 \times 11^0$

Kit. $12^{10} \times 12^0$

R.

P.

DN

Br. 3 $11^0 \times 11^0$

LIN.

W.

D.

Din. $11^0 \times 14^0$

10'-0" CLG.

E.

LIN.

WHIRLPOOL

Mbr. $14^0 \times 15^0$

10'-0" CLG.

SHELVES

Gar. $23^4 \times 22^4$

COVERED PORCH

56' - 0"

55' - 4"

© design basics inc.

The covered porch adds a classic touch to the elevation with repeating arch-topped windows and columns.

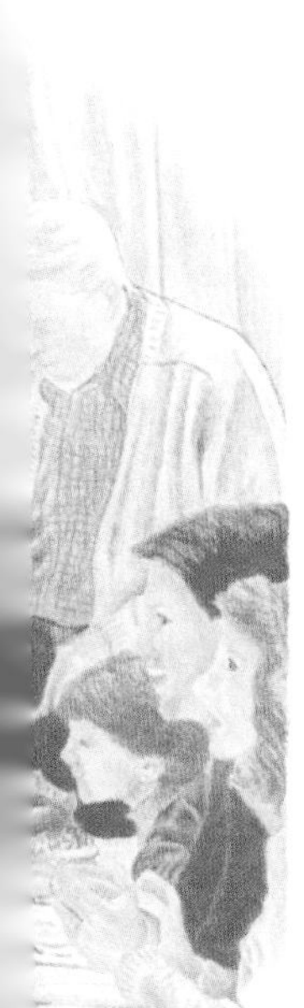

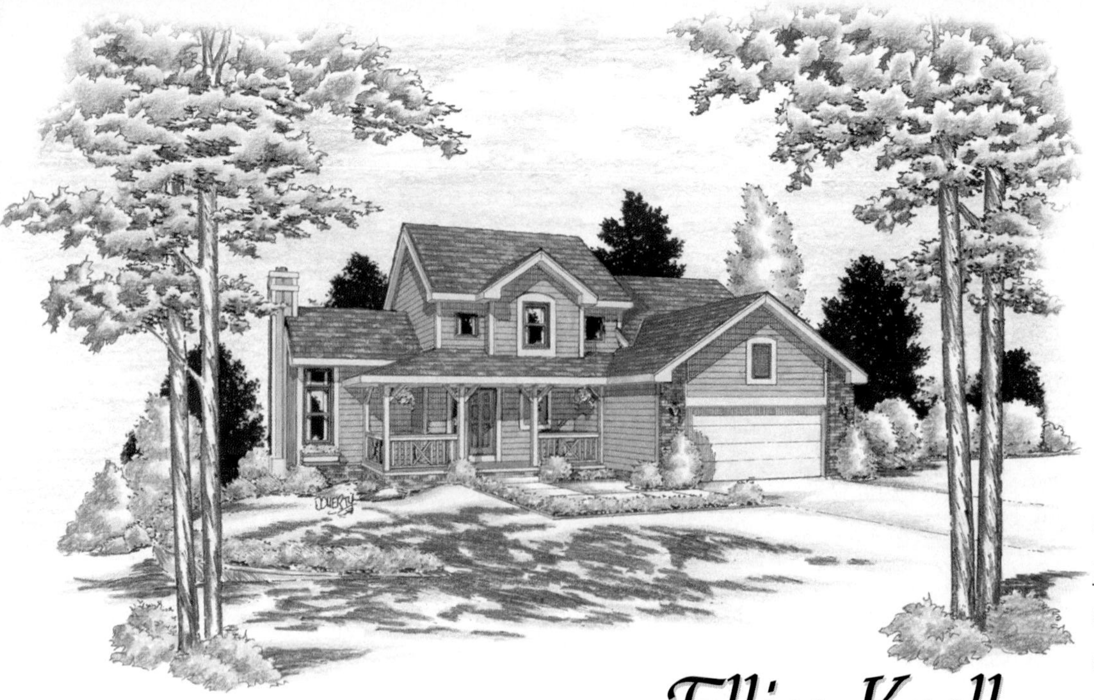

> *My life holds its meaning in these memories, in the roots of my family... we anticipate building a new home – a new place to house my roots.*

welcome, but also nurture. It must genuinely enrich the lives of those who enter and leave them with a piece of itself to take along. It must naturally foster new memories. It must cling to them and hold them as dearly as I do. It must grow young in spirit along with us as we age. It must be a place that my children (and eventually, my grandchildren) will fondly recall as a part of their legacy. It must reinvent itself as our family and friends change. It must be large. It must make room for my roots. ◆

Ellies Knoll

#28A-8027 Plan Price $395

Main Floor:	1210 Sq. Ft.
Second Floor:	405 Sq. Ft.
Total Square Feet:	1615 Sq. Ft.

Br. 3 10²x 11⁰
Br. 2 10²x 11⁰
L.
L.
DN
OPEN TO BELOW

The upstairs bedrooms are serviced by a hall bath with dual lavs and compartmented stool and tub.

A secluded entrance to the master suite ensures privacy from the living areas.

Entertaining is enhanced by a flowing arrangement between the entry, great room and kitchen area.

The covered front porch offers a quaint welcome to friends as well as a shady retreat to unwind.

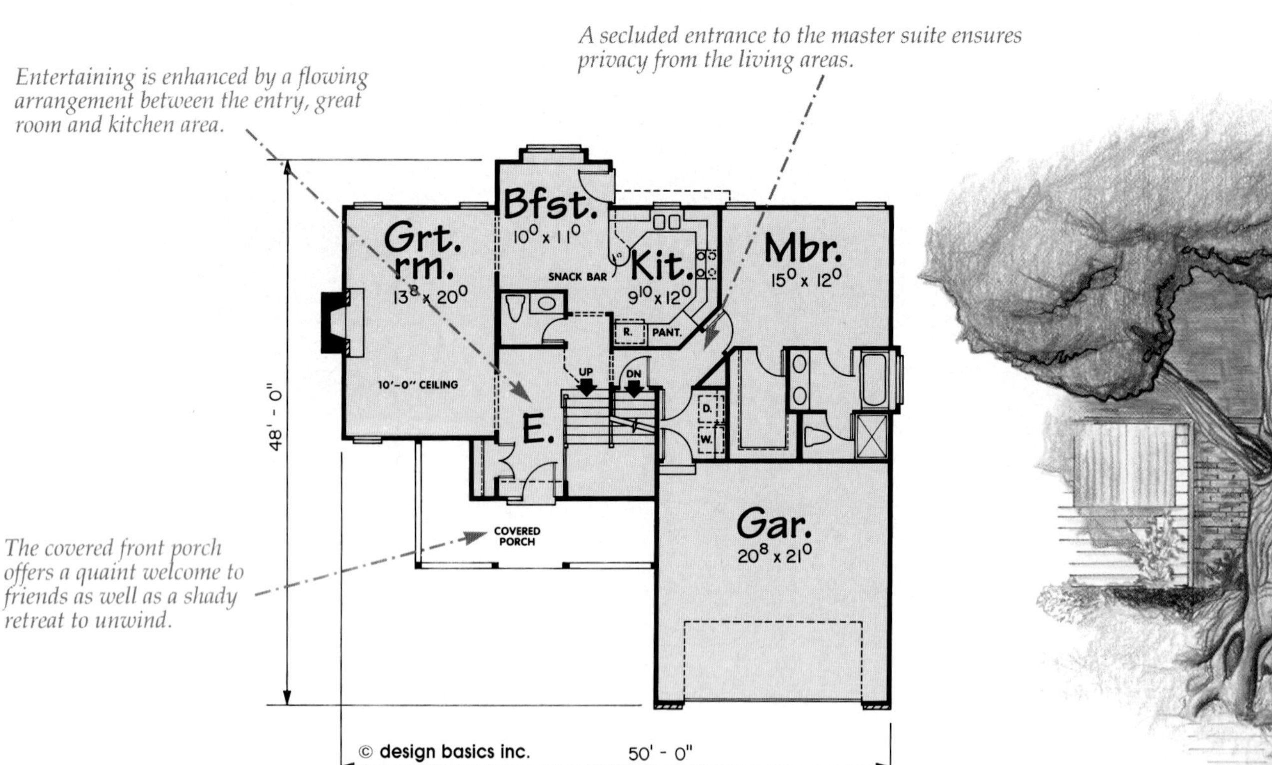

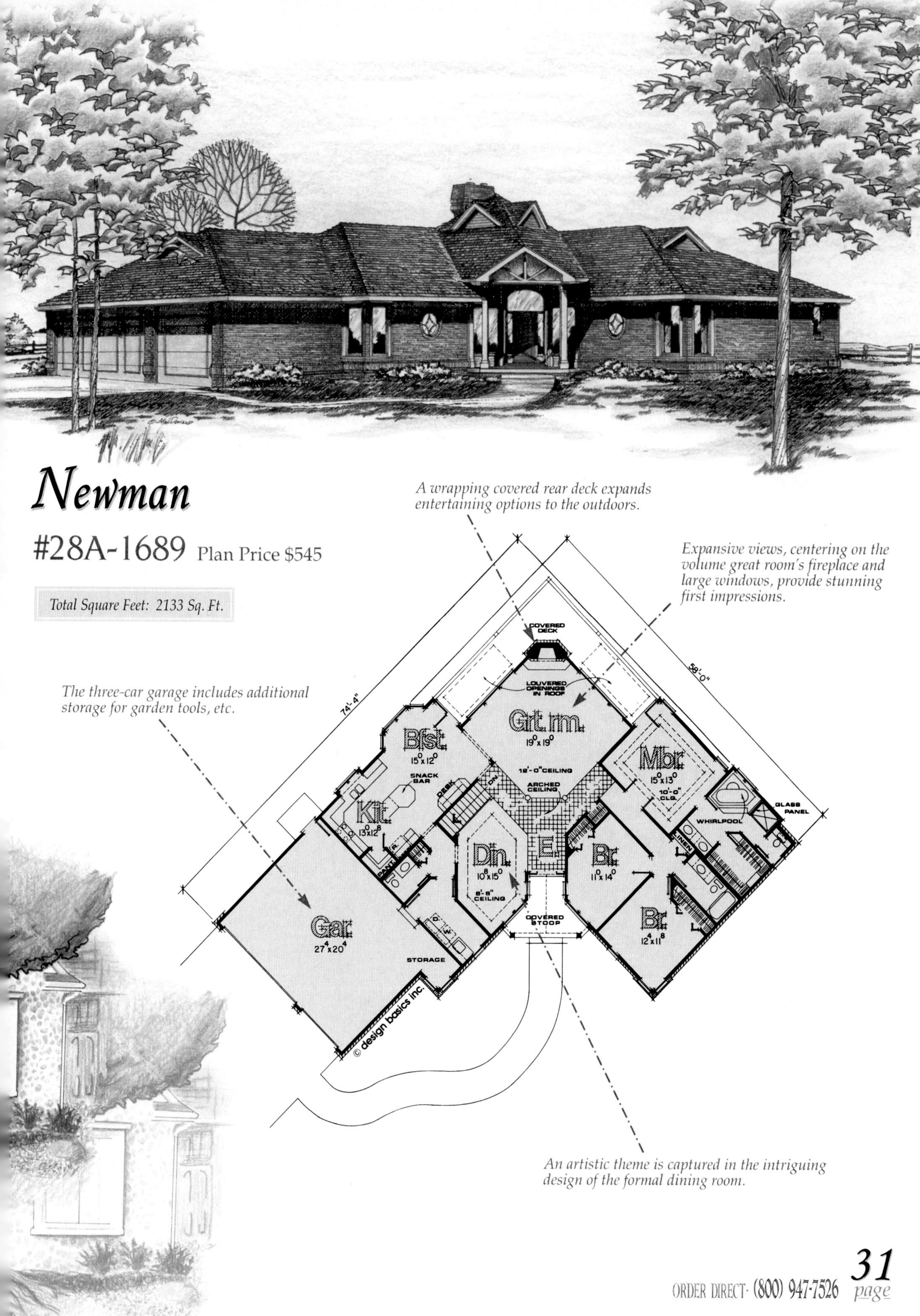

Newman

#28A-1689 Plan Price $545

Total Square Feet: 2133 Sq. Ft.

A wrapping covered rear deck expands entertaining options to the outdoors.

Expansive views, centering on the volume great room's fireplace and large windows, provide stunning first impressions.

The three-car garage includes additional storage for garden tools, etc.

An artistic theme is captured in the intriguing design of the formal dining room.

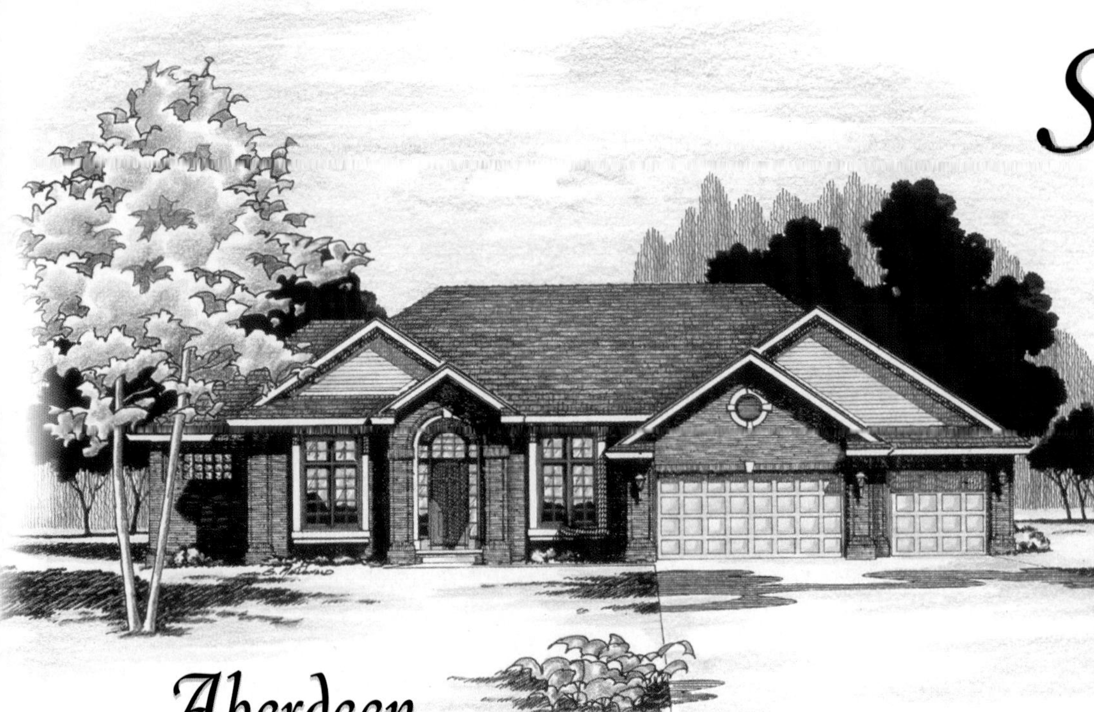

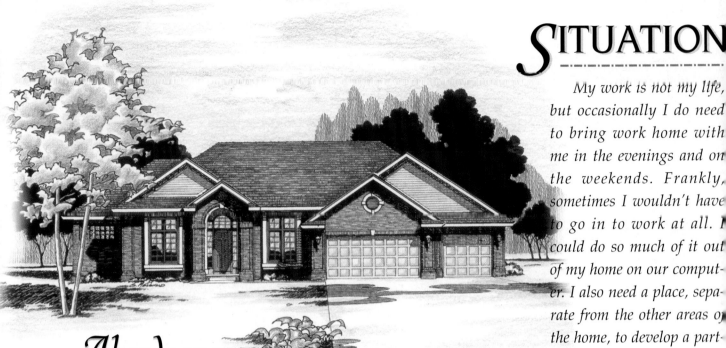

Aberdeen

#28A-2321 Plan Price $555

Total Square Feet: 2276 Sq. Ft.

Tall windows brighten the breakfast area and kitchen.

TRANSOMS · Bfst. 13⁰ x 11⁰ · TRANSOMS · Grt. rm. 16⁰ x 19⁸ · 9'-4" CEILINGS · WET BAR · SNACK BAR · DESK · Mbr. 13⁰ x 15⁵ · DRESSER/ ENT. CENTER · Kit. 13⁰ x 10⁵ · Br. 2 12⁰ x 11⁰ · Br. 3 12⁰ x 11⁶ · DN · LIN. · W. D. · WHIRL-POOL · GLASS BLOCK · Den 13³ x 13³ · 10'-8" CEILING · E. · Din. 13⁰ x 13⁷ · 10'-8" CEILING · Gar. 31³ x 23⁸ · COVERED STOOP · TRANSOMS · 56'-0" · 72'-0"

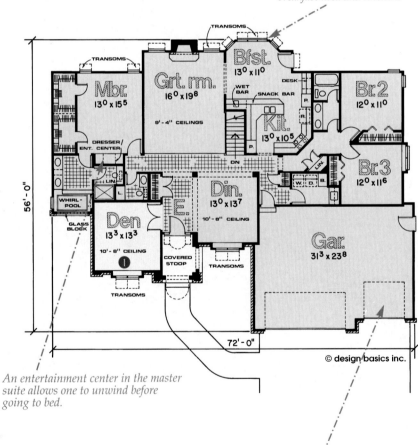

© design basics inc.

An entertainment center in the master suite allows one to unwind before going to bed.

A third stall makes the perfect place for a golf cart or riding lawnmower.

SITUATION

My work is not my life, but occasionally I do need to bring work home with me in the evenings and on the weekends. Frankly, sometimes I wouldn't have to go in to work at all. I could do so much of it out of my home on our computer. I also need a place, separate from the other areas of the home, to develop a part-time home business we're thinking about launching soon. If only we had a place to work. . .

SOLUTION

Both the Aberdeen and the Douglas have excellent options for a home office. Just inside the Aberdeen, double doors lead to a den that's secluded from the rest of the home (❶, at left). Another great place for an office is the loft in the Douglas (❷, at right). It features a window to the back and a view overlooking the family room.

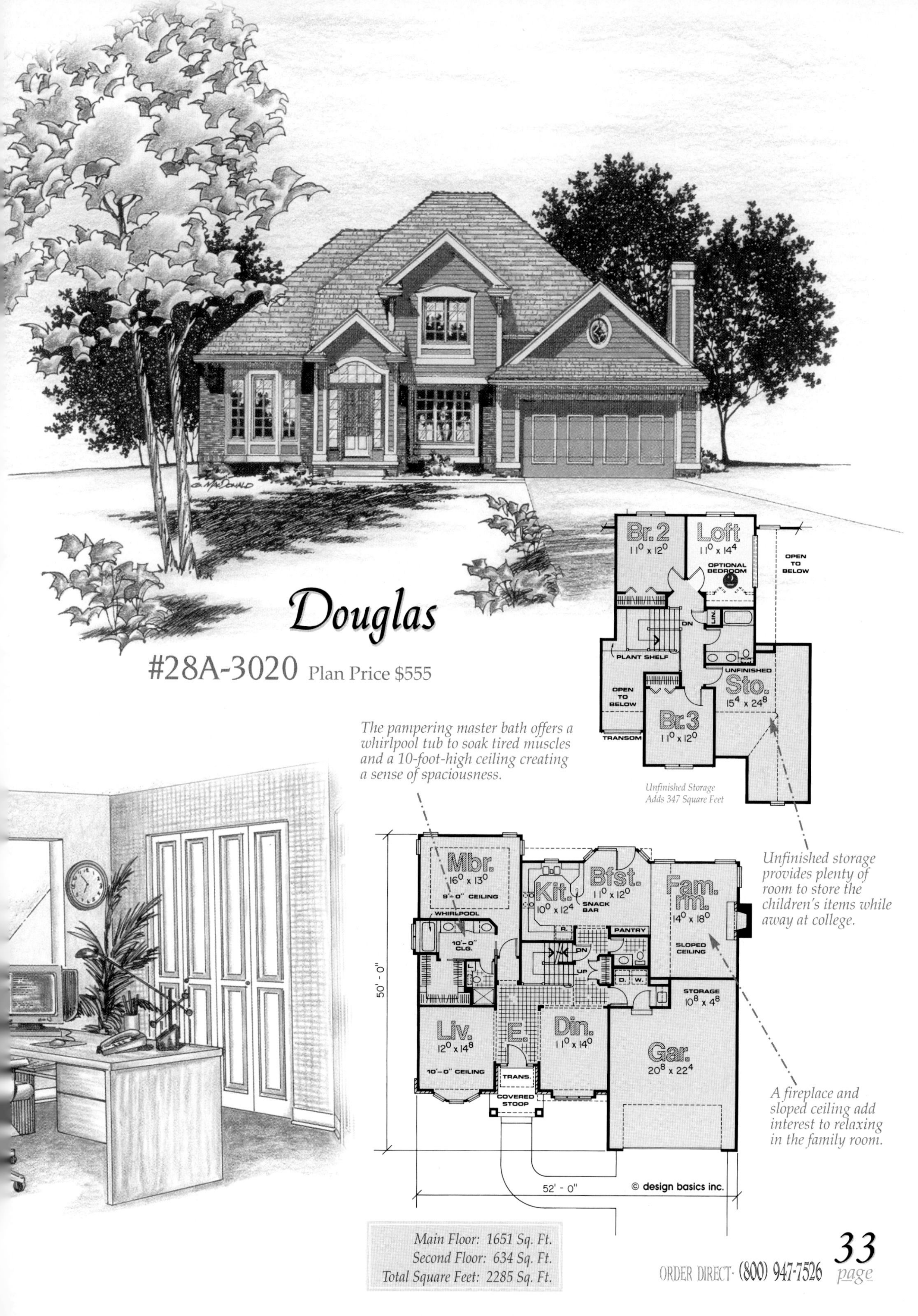

Douglas

#28A-3020 Plan Price $555

The pampering master bath offers a whirlpool tub to soak tired muscles and a 10-foot-high ceiling creating a sense of spaciousness.

Unfinished Storage Adds 347 Square Feet

Unfinished storage provides plenty of room to store the children's items while away at college.

A fireplace and sloped ceiling add interest to relaxing in the family room.

Main Floor: 1651 Sq. Ft.
Second Floor: 634 Sq. Ft.
Total Square Feet: 2285 Sq. Ft.

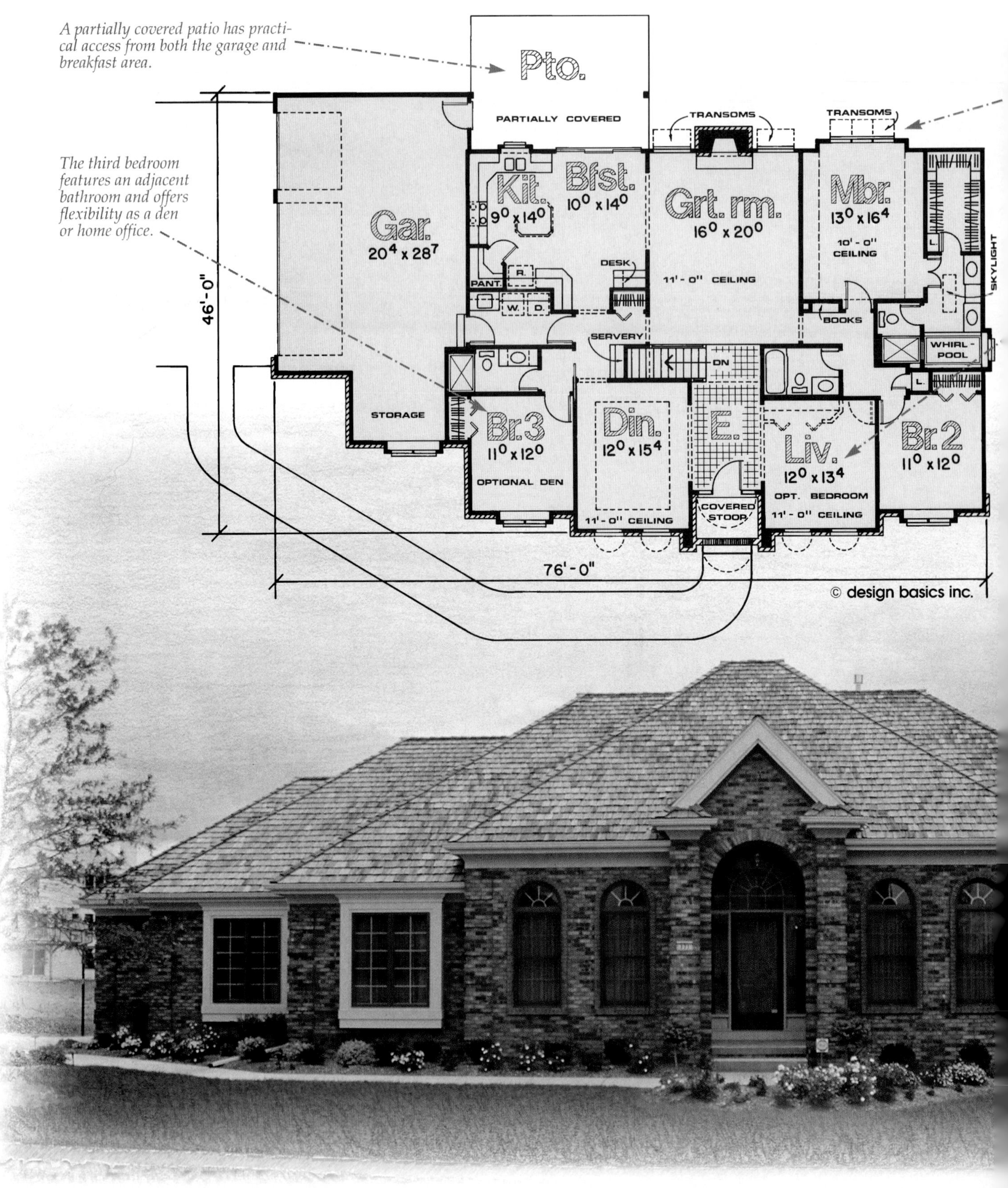

Greensboro

#28A-2326 Plan Price $545

PHOTO BY: DESIGN BASICS INC.
BUILT BY: TWEEDT ENGINEERING AND CONSTRUCTION

The home in the photograph may be altered from the original pla

Large windows brighten the master suite with double doors that open to a luxurious bath area.

The versatile living room can easily convert into a fourth bedroom.

Total Square Feet: 2172 Sq. Ft.

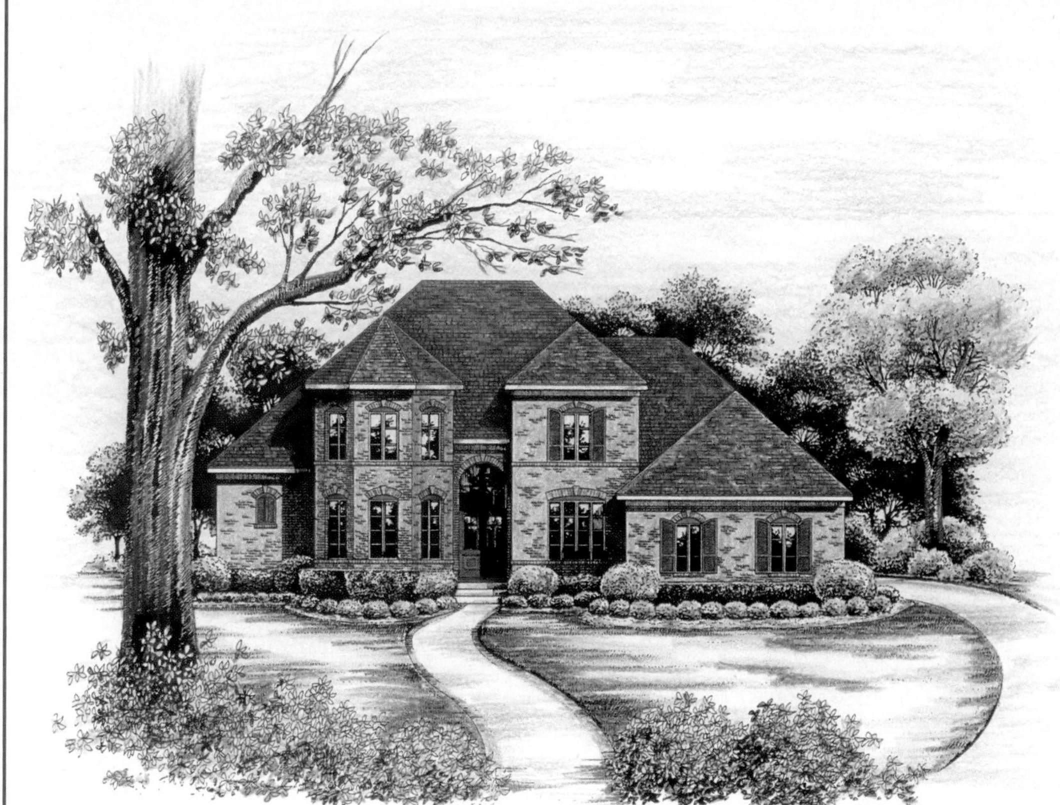

Woodlands Showcase

#28A-9160 Plan Price $660

Main Floor: 1906 Sq. Ft.
Second Floor: 749 Sq. Ft.
Total Square Feet: 2655 Sq. Ft.

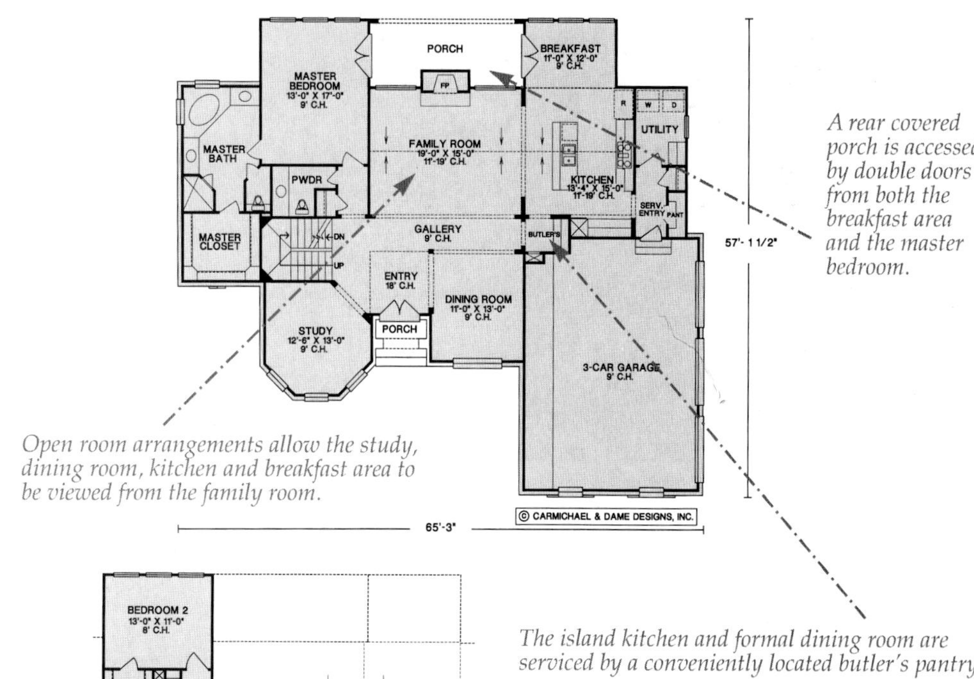

A rear covered porch is accessed by double doors from both the breakfast area and the master bedroom.

Open room arrangements allow the study, dining room, kitchen and breakfast area to be viewed from the family room.

The island kitchen and formal dining room are serviced by a conveniently located butler's pantry.

A second-level balcony provides dramatic views overlooking the family room and entry below.

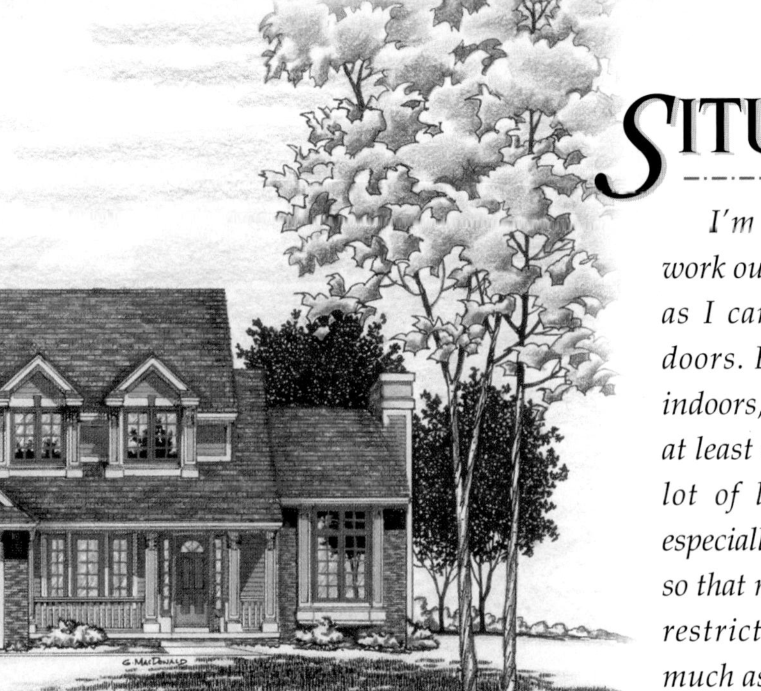

SITUATION

I'm a nature freak. I work outdoors and as much as I can, I try to be outdoors. Even if I have to be indoors, I want to be able to at least see nature. I want a lot of light coming in – especially in the living areas so that my home doesn't feel restricted or dark. And as much as I hate to admit the fact that I'm getting older, a lot of light helps me to see better. Plain and simple, I want a lot of windows in my home. . .

An island counter helps organize the kitchen.

A 10-foot ceiling adds volume to the master bath.

A large porch welcomes the addition of a bench to relax upon.

© design basics inc.

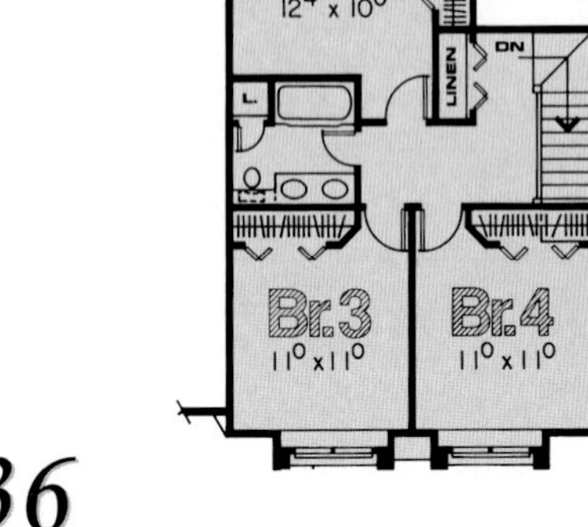

SOLUTION

Spectacular windows highlight the living areas of the Hawthorne. The kitchen, breakfast area and gathering room (❶, at right and interior view) offer an abundance of natural light through window upon window lining the rear. Arched windows brighten the breakfast area in the Eldridge. Nearby, the great room also features views to the front and rear (❷, at left).

Eldridge

#28A-3064 Plan Price $535

Main Floor: 1414 Sq. Ft.
Second Floor: 641 Sq. Ft.
Total Square Feet: 2055 Sq. Ft.

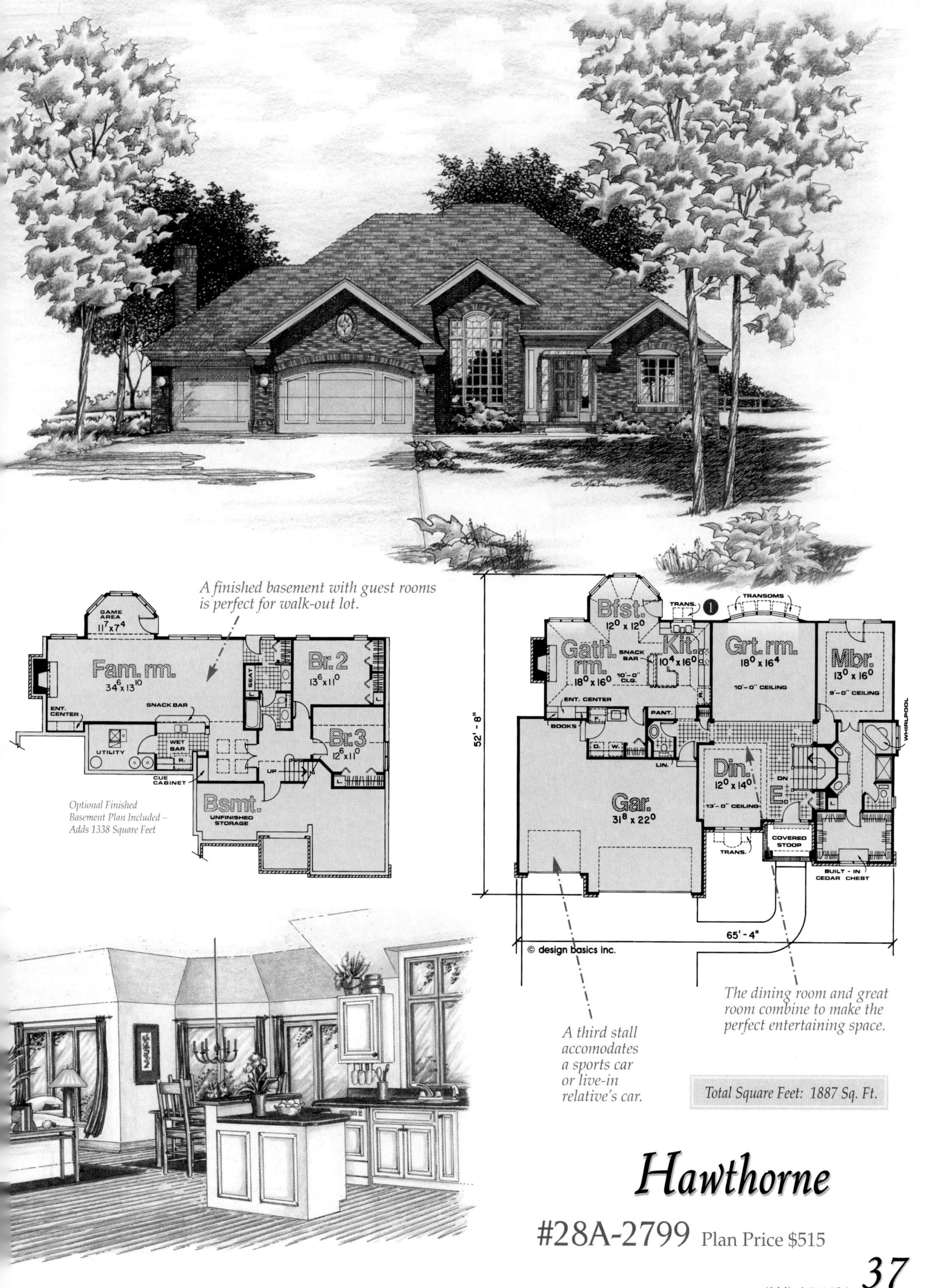

A finished basement with guest rooms is perfect for walk-out lot.
GAME AREA 11⁷x7⁴
Fam. rm. 34⁶x13¹⁰
Br. 2 13⁶x11⁰
Br. 3 12⁶x11⁰
SEAT
ENT. CENTER
SNACK BAR
UTILITY
WET BAR
CUE CABINET
UP
Bsmt. UNFINISHED STORAGE
Optional Finished Basement Plan Included – Adds 1338 Square Feet
Bfst. 12⁰ x 12⁰
TRANS.
TRANSOMS
Gath. rm. 18⁰ x 16⁰
SNACK BAR
10'-0" CLG.
Kit. 10⁴ x 16⁰
Grt. rm. 18⁰ x 16⁴
10'-0" CEILING
Mbr. 13⁰ x 16⁰
9'-0" CEILING
WHIRLPOOL
ENT. CENTER
BOOKS
PANT.
LIN.
Din. 12⁰ x 14⁰
13'-0" CEILING
DN
E.
Gar. 31⁸ x 22⁰
TRANS.
COVERED STOOP
BUILT - IN CEDAR CHEST
52' - 8"
65' - 4"
© design basics inc.
A third stall accomodates a sports car or live-in relative's car.
The dining room and great room combine to make the perfect entertaining space.

Total Square Feet: 1887 Sq. Ft.

Hawthorne

#28A-2799 Plan Price $515

SITUATION

Even though our kids are finally gone – one off to college and the other in the armed services – we're still stuck with storing their "things" until they're finished with their degrees. (It amazes us how much they've accumulated in 18 years!) We'd like to be able to change their bedrooms into guest rooms or a much-needed office, but we need much more storage space in our home before we can do that. . .

SOLUTION

The Sayler and Silver Springs both offer large storage areas or "bonus rooms" on the second floor (❶, at right and ❷, at far right). Each area is large enough to store seasonal items, family keepsakes, as well as the childrens' things until they move out permanently. They are also great places to think about finishing into extra living space .

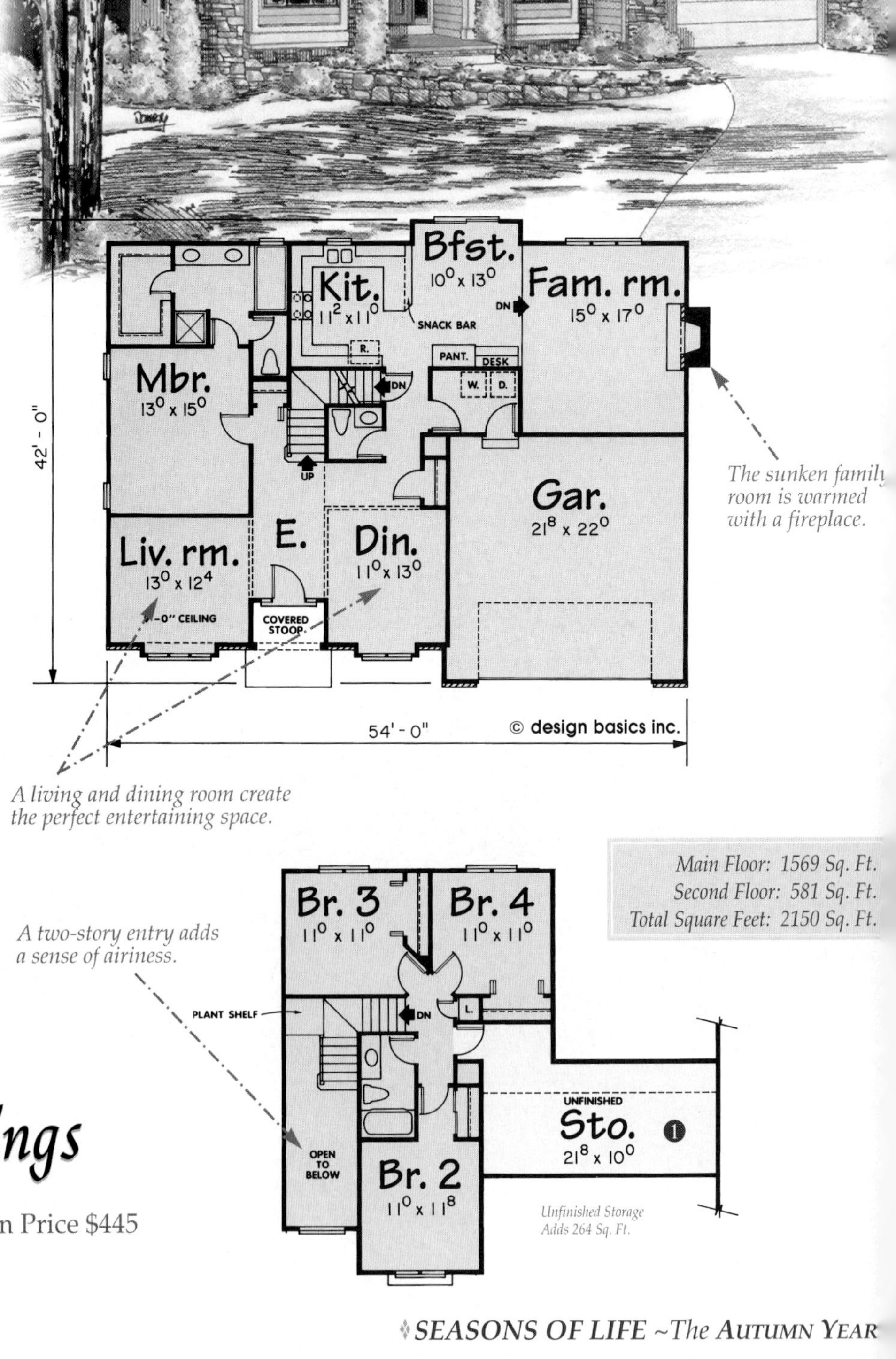

The sunken family room is warmed with a fireplace.

A living and dining room create the perfect entertaining space.

A two-story entry adds a sense of airiness.

Unfinished Storage Adds 264 Sq. Ft.

Main Floor: 1569 Sq. Ft.
Second Floor: 581 Sq. Ft.
Total Square Feet: 2150 Sq. Ft.

Silver Springs

#28A-8124 Plan Price $445

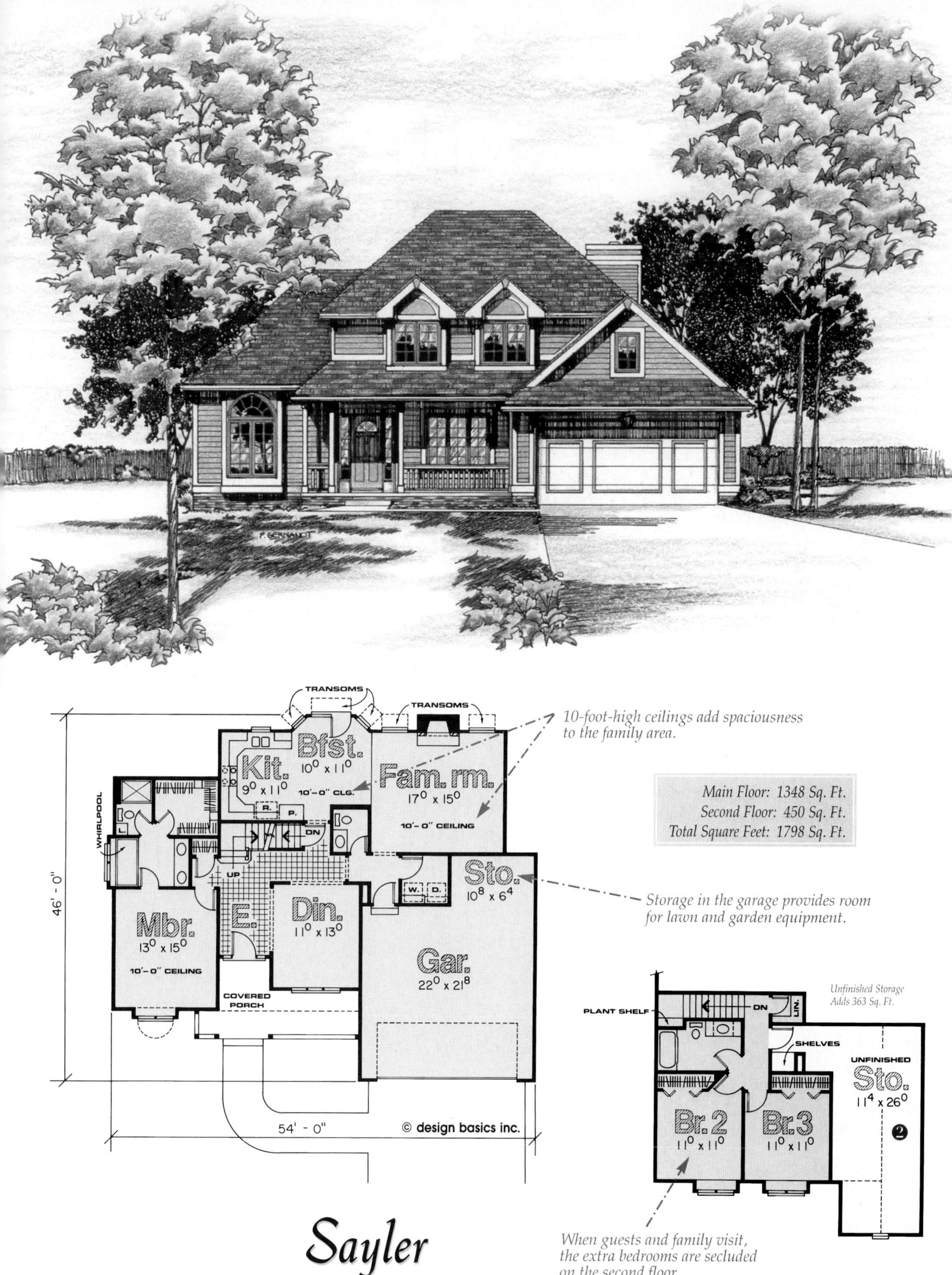

F. BERNARDT
TRANSOMS
TRANSOMS
10-foot-high ceilings add spaciousness to the family area.
Bfst.
10⁰ x 11⁰
Kit.
9⁰ x 11⁰
10'-0" CLG.
Fam. rm.
17⁰ x 15⁰
10'-0" CEILING
R.
P.
DN
WHIRLPOOL
L.
UP
W.
D.
Sto.
10⁸ x 6⁴
Storage in the garage provides room for lawn and garden equipment.
Main Floor: 1348 Sq. Ft.
Second Floor: 450 Sq. Ft.
Total Square Feet: 1798 Sq. Ft.
46' - 0"
Mbr.
13⁰ x 15⁰
10'-0" CEILING
E.
Din.
11⁰ x 13⁰
Gar.
22⁰ x 21⁸
COVERED PORCH
54' - 0"
© design basics inc.
Unfinished Storage Adds 363 Sq. Ft.
PLANT SHELF
DN
LIN.
SHELVES
UNFINISHED
Sto.
11⁴ x 26⁰
Br. 2
11⁰ x 11⁰
Br. 3
11⁰ x 11⁰
When guests and family visit, the extra bedrooms are secluded on the second floor.
Sayler

#28A-3076 Plan Price $505

OPEN KITCHEN AREAS . . . *Name the most important part of a home and inevitably many will mention the kitchen. Today's kitchens have been transformed from working spaces solely, to also functioning as living spaces – often where the family gathers together informally. The following plans feature kitchens that function both ways.*

PRACTICAL PANTRY

Main Floor: 1697 Sq. Ft.
Second Floor: 694 Sq. Ft.
Total Square Feet: 2391 Sq. Ft.

Ashton

#28A-2203 Plan Price $565

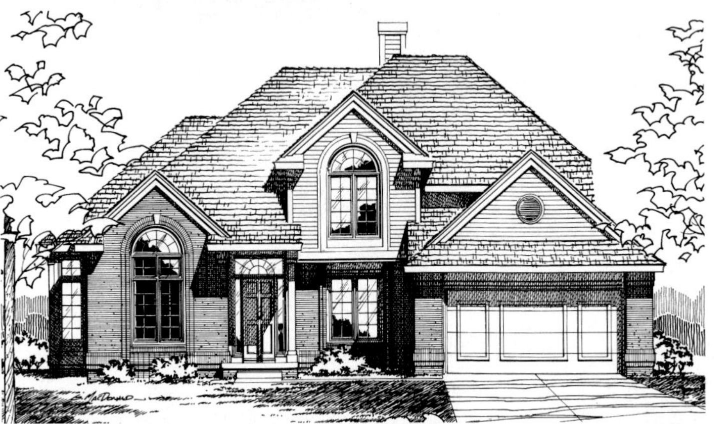

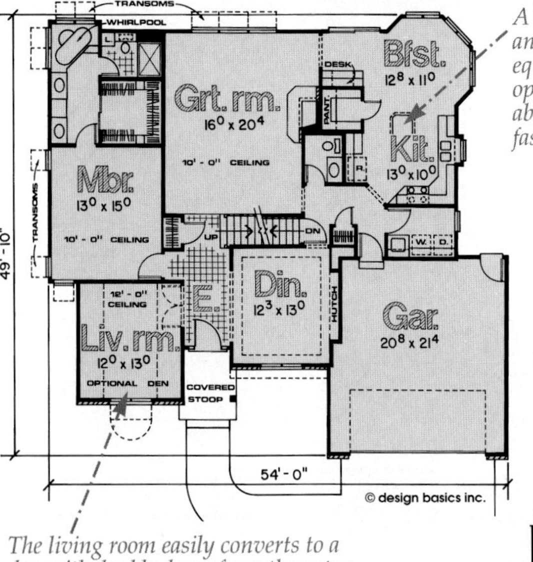

A walk-in pantry and island counter equip this kitchen, open to a comfortable sunny breakfast area.

The living room easily converts to a den with double doors from the entry.

Built-in desks benefit all three secondary bedrooms.

Br. 2
13⁴ x 11⁰
DESK
DN
Br. 4
11⁰ x 12⁰
Br. 3
11³ x 12⁰
10' - 0" CEILING

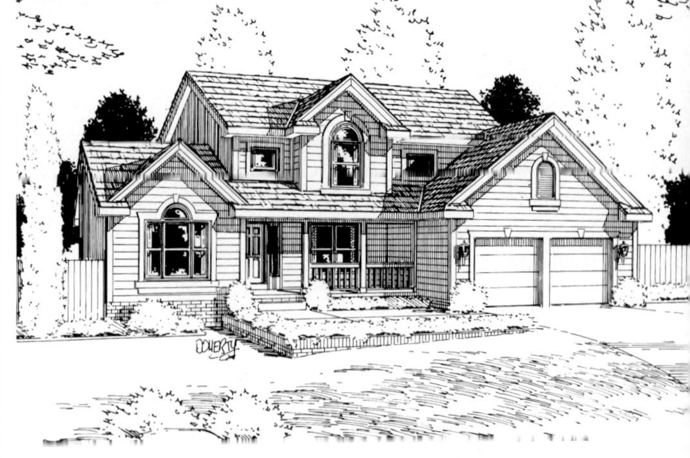

FOR THE SERIOUS CHEF

Main Floor: 1505 Sq. Ft.
Second Floor: 610 Sq. Ft.
Total Square Feet: 2115 Sq. Ft.

Kerry Crossing

#28A-8054 Plan Price $445

An L-shaped island counter and bayed windows complement a kitchen/dinette area that is open and unrestricted.

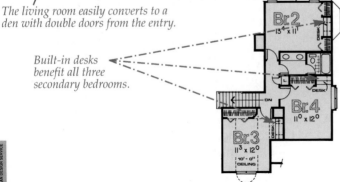

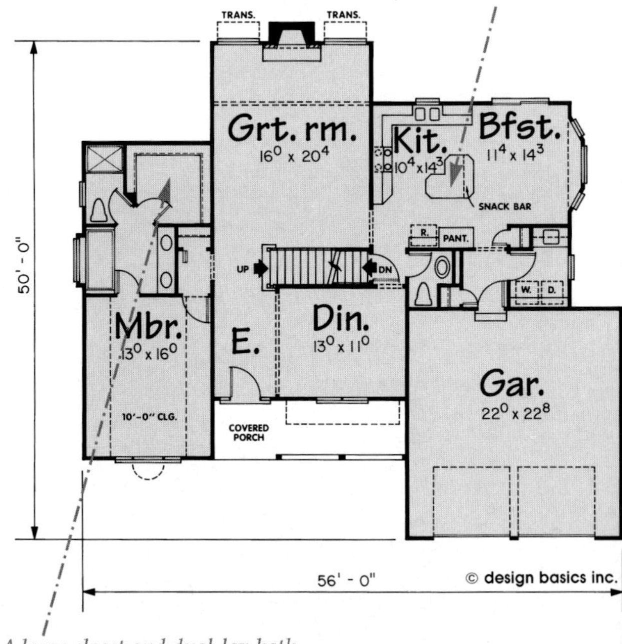

A large closet and dual-lav bath serve the master suite.

Twin closets frame an arched window in bedroom #2.

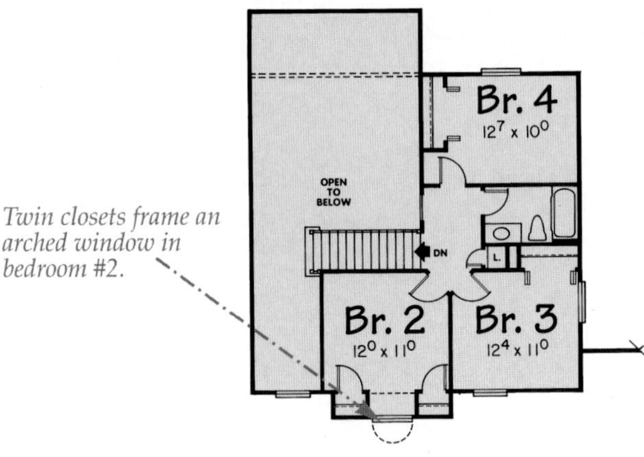

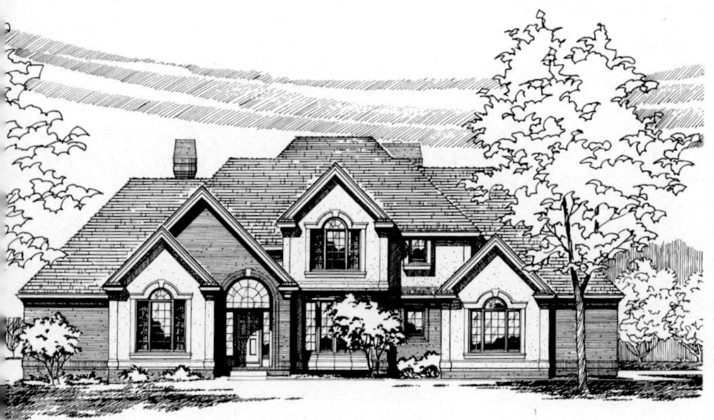

COMFORTABLE HEARTH ROOM

Main Floor: 2252 Sq. Ft.
Second Floor: 920 Sq. Ft.
Total Square Feet: 3172 Sq. Ft.

Normandy

#28A-2249 Plan Price $645

A stylish breakfast area and comfortable hearth room are linked with an organized kitchen for everyday living.

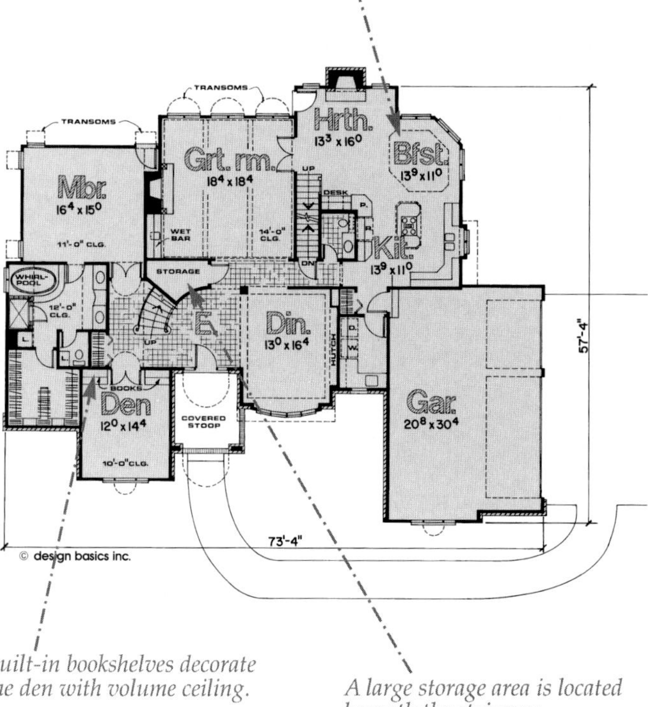

Built-in bookshelves decorate the den with volume ceiling.

A large storage area is located beneath the stairway.

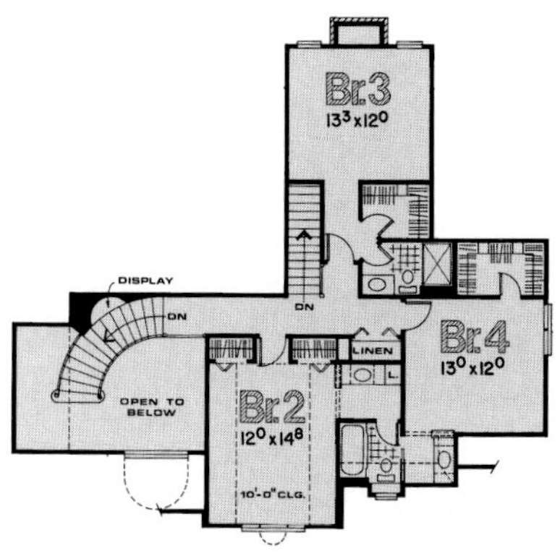

PAMPERING KITCHEN PANTRY

Main Floor: 1860 Sq. Ft.
Second Floor: 848 Sq. Ft.
Total Square Feet: 2708 Sq. Ft.

Cordeaux

#28A-2174 Plan Price $605

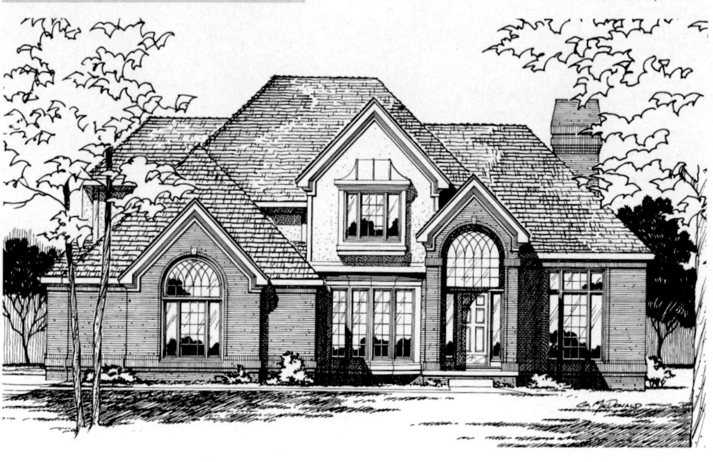

Bayed windows illuminate the island kitchen with corner pantry.

A see-thru fireplace with built-in entertainment shelves warms the family and living rooms.

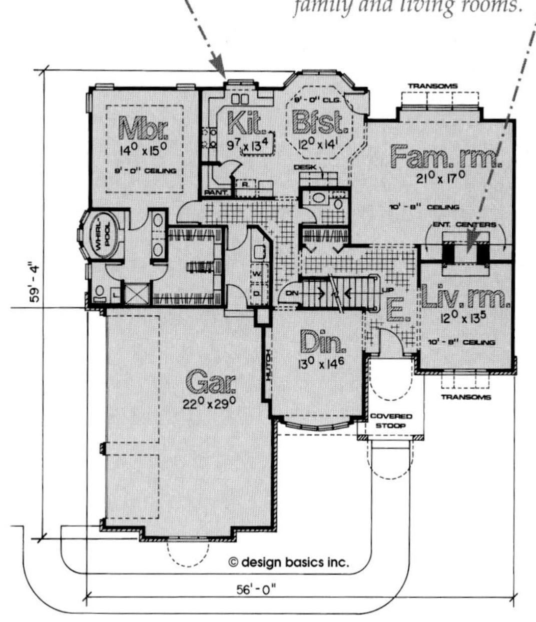

A walk-in linen closet provides extra storage on the second floor.

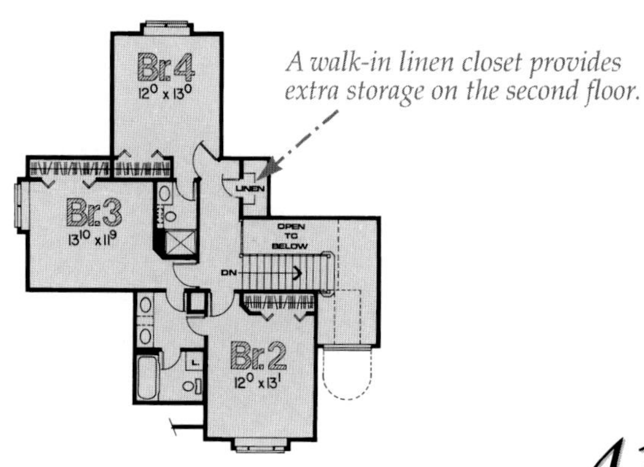

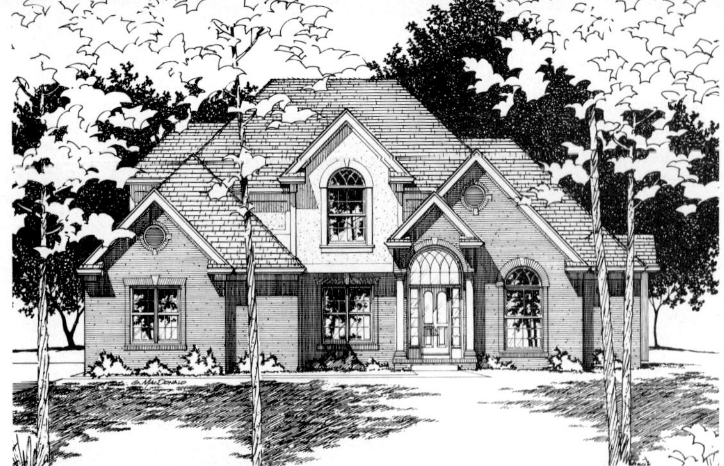

VIEW'S TO THE GREAT ROOM

Main Floor: 1777 Sq. Ft.
Second Floor: 719 Sq. Ft.
Total Square Feet: 2496 Sq. Ft.

Pinnacle

#28A-3284 Plan Price $575

The sunken great room is open to both the entry and kitchen/breakfast area.

Bayed windows complement the master suite featuring a sloped ceiling and whirlpool.

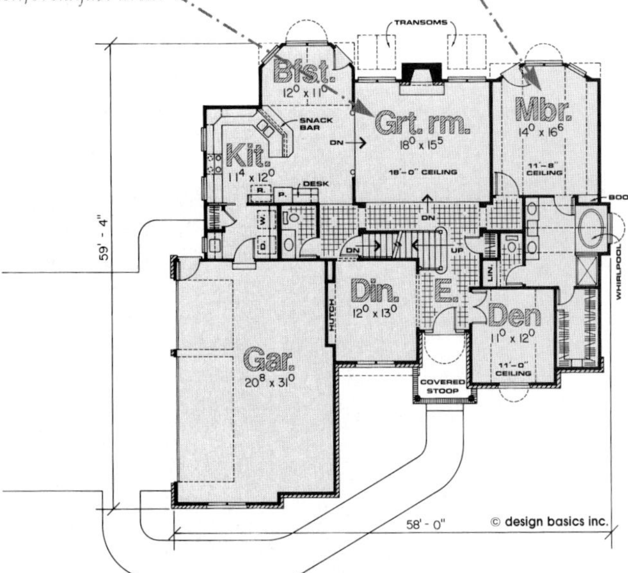

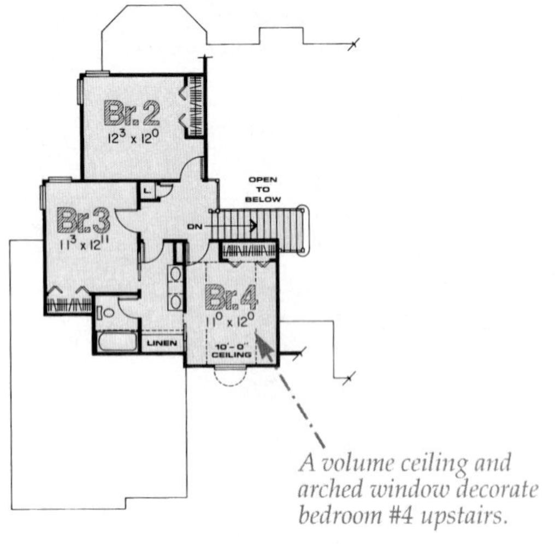

A volume ceiling and arched window decorate bedroom #4 upstairs.

ARRANGED TO ENTERTAIN

Main Floor: 1595 Sq. Ft.
Second Floor: 641 Sq. Ft.
Total Square Feet: 2236 Sq. Ft.

Kentbrook

#28A-2176 Plan Price $555

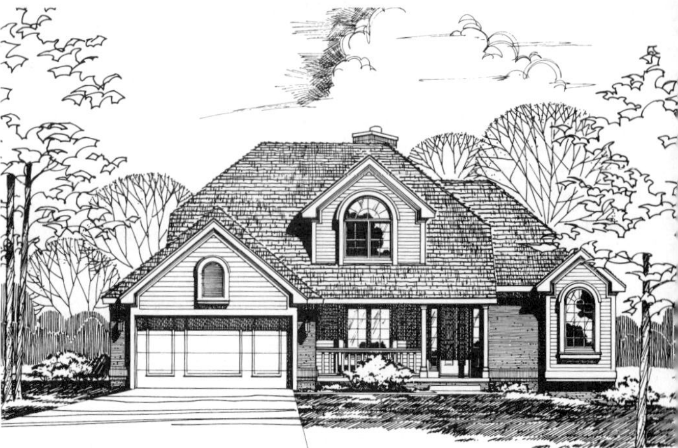

The layout of the island kitchen, open to the breakfast area and hearth room, helps create the ambiance of one large comfortable living space.

An angled see-thru f place is shared betwe the great room and bayed hearth room.

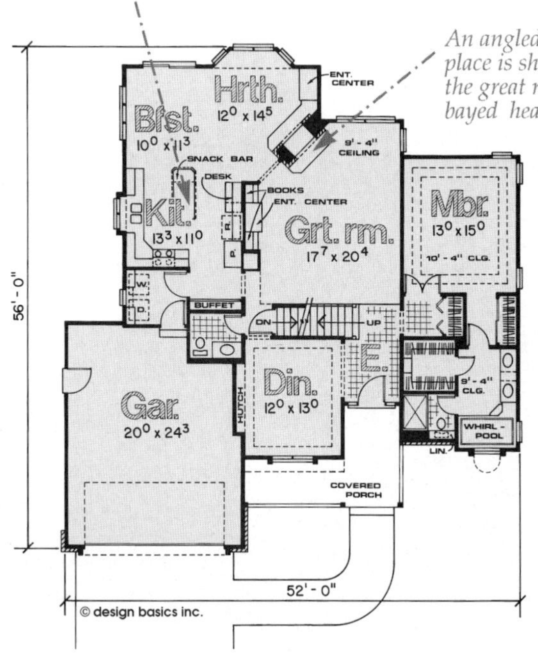

The built-in desk in be room #2 is enhanced b sloped ceiling.

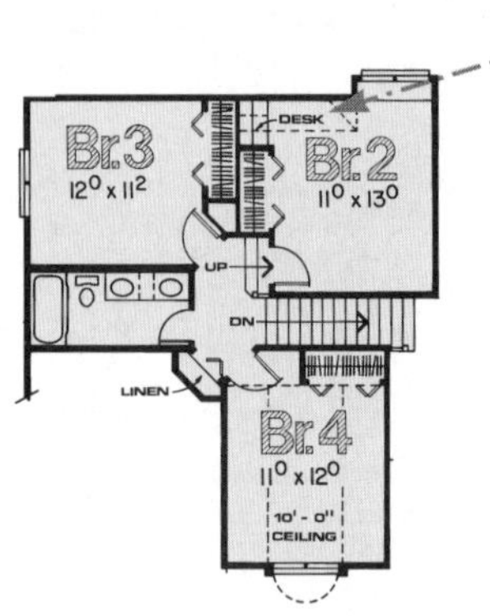

DEFINED FAMILY AREA

Main Floor: 1174 Sq. Ft.
Second Floor: 372 Sq. Ft.
Total Square Feet: 1546 Sq. Ft.

Jenkins

#28A-3464 Plan Price $485

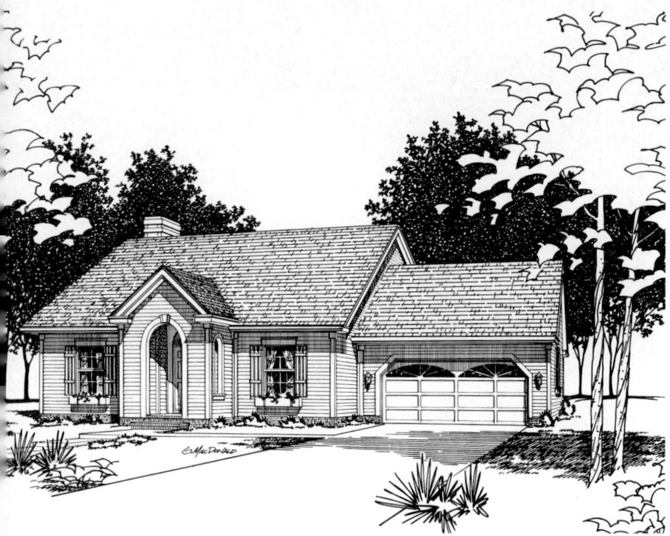

The family room, accented with a cathedral ceiling and three windows, completes a defined family area at the rear of the home.

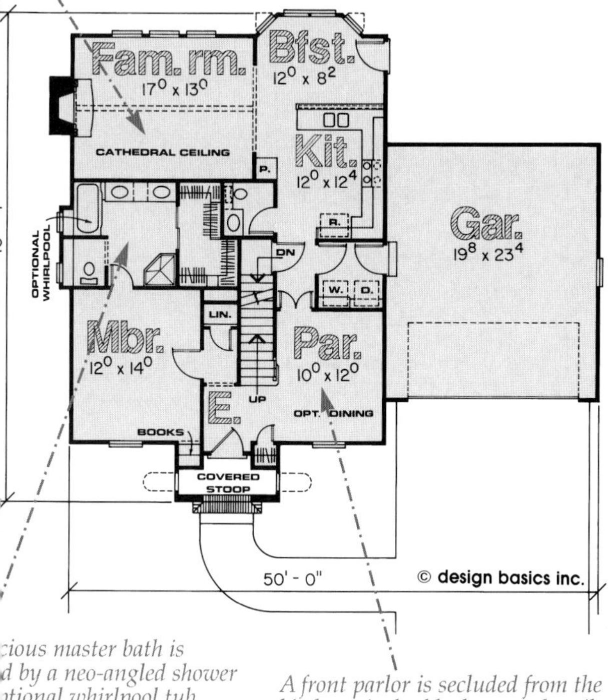

…cious master bath is …d by a neo-angled shower …tional whirlpool tub.

A front parlor is secluded from the kitchen via double doors and easily converts into a dining room.

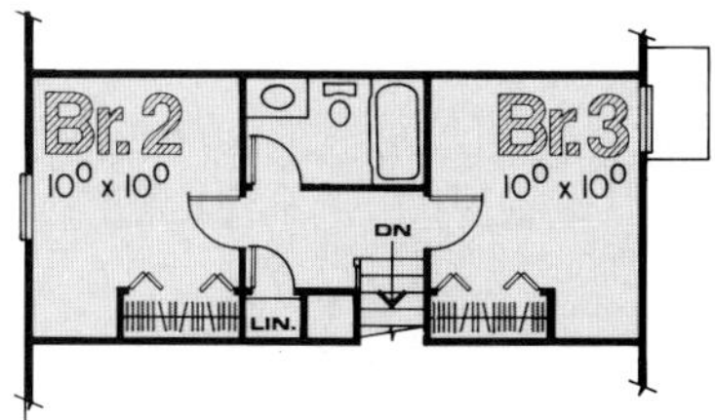

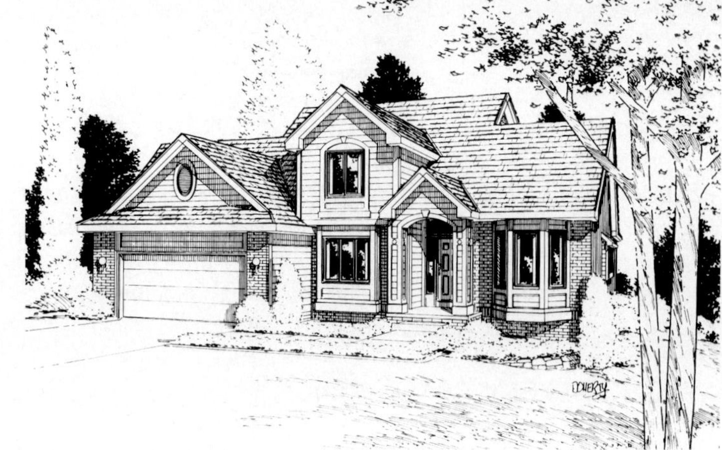

CONVENIENT CONNECTION

Main Floor: 1651 Sq. Ft.
Second Floor: 639 Sq. Ft.
Total Square Feet: 2290 Sq. Ft.

Barretts Bend

#28A-8036 Plan Price $455

A cathedral ceiling centering on a fireplace enhances the family room.

A large pantry and bayed windows provide convenience and light to the nearby kitchen.

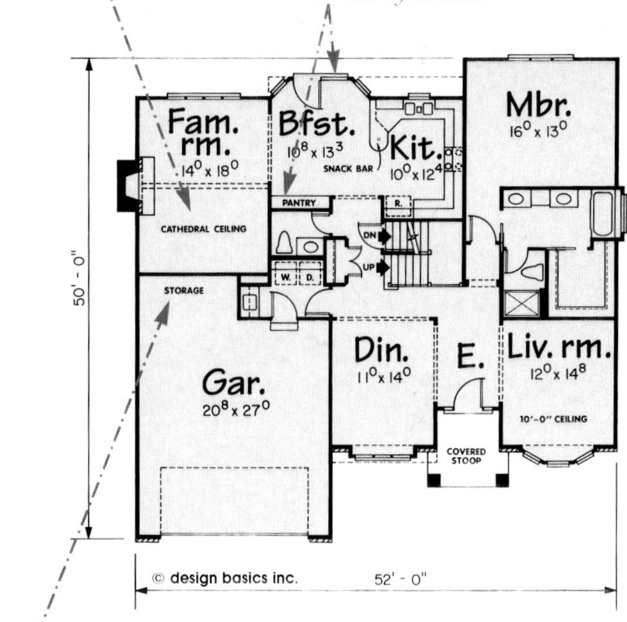

Storage space in the garage leaves room for tools and lawn equipment.

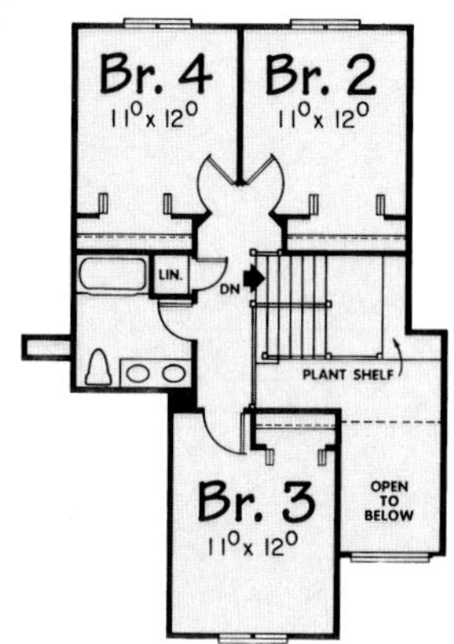

Memorable Master Suites . . .

One of the most relaxing things about any home is the bath area. Whether it be a soaking tub, where we unwind or a large vanity where we take our time getting ready, the perfect master suites are those that are a retreat in and of themselves. You're sure to find a master suite for you among the following plans.

Privately Pampering

Main Floor: 2041 Sq. Ft.
Second Floor: 809 Sq. Ft.
Total Square Feet: 2850 Sq. Ft.

Thornhill

#28A-3494 Plan Price $615

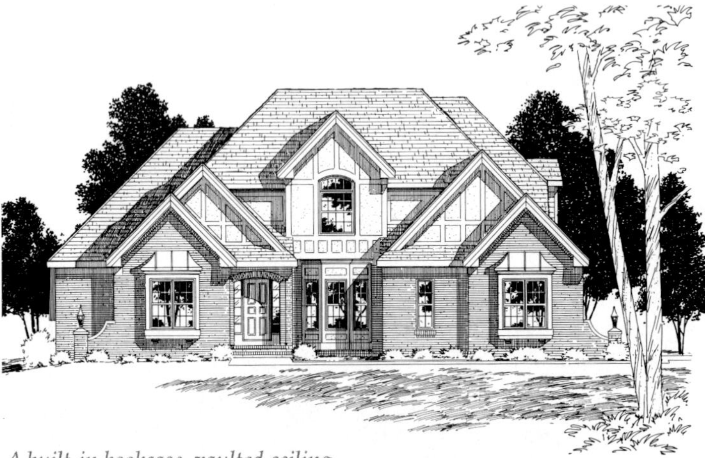

A built-in bookcase, vaulted ceiling and door to the back enhance the relaxing master bedroom.

A hallway just off the entry secludes the master suite and den in privacy.

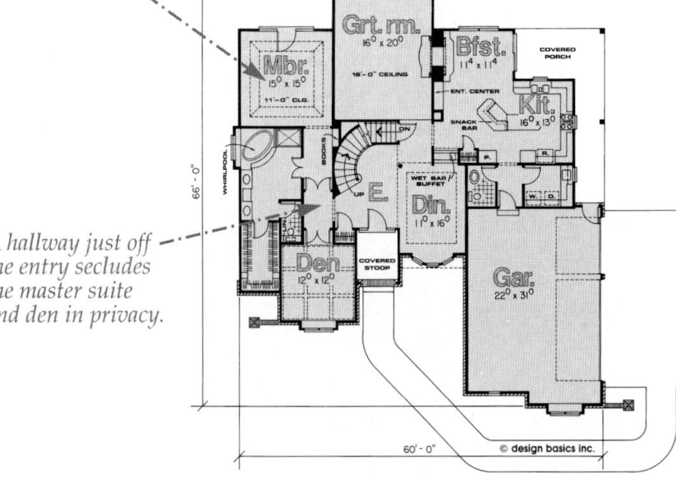

The dramatic great room can be viewed from a second-floor balcony.

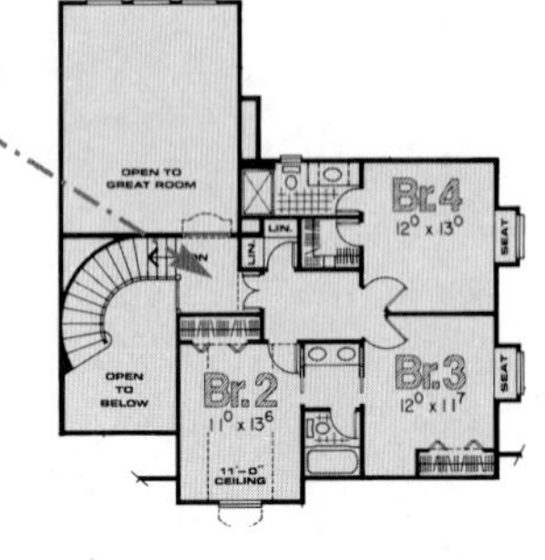

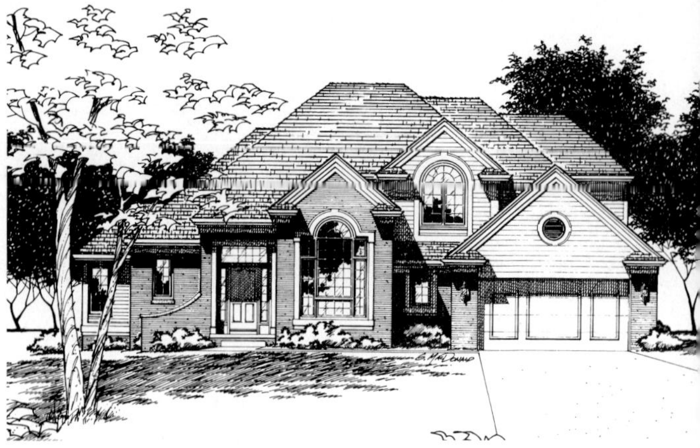

Angles for Intrigue

Main Floor: 1518 Sq. Ft.
Second Floor: 697 Sq. Ft.
Total Square Feet: 2215 Sq. Ft.

Bentley

#28A-2828 Plan Price $555

A corner whirlpool tub and neo-angled shower are showcased behind French doors in the master bath.

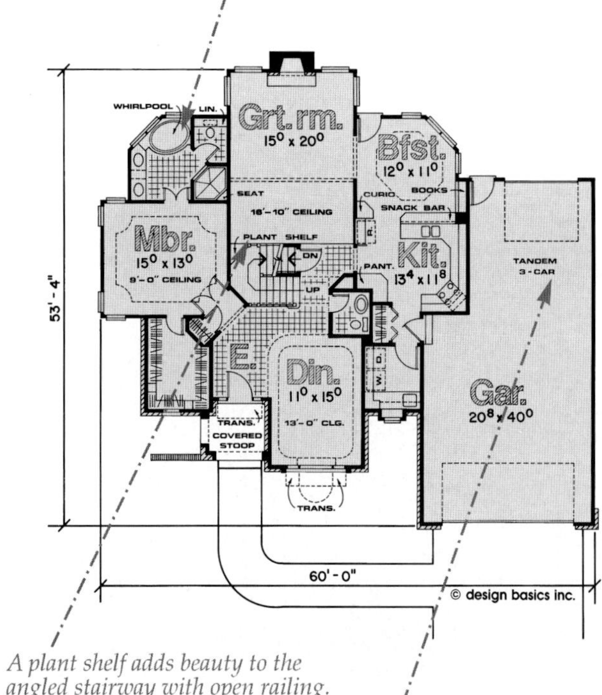

A plant shelf adds beauty to the angled stairway with open railing.

A three-car tandem garage provides convenient access to an alley or golf course.

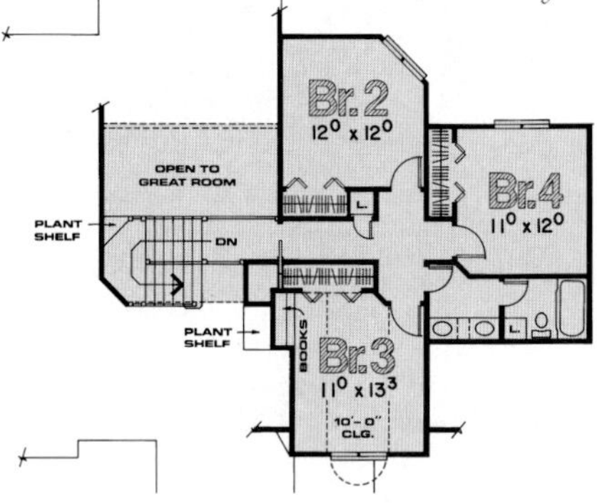

design basics inc. HOME PLAN DESIGN SERVICE

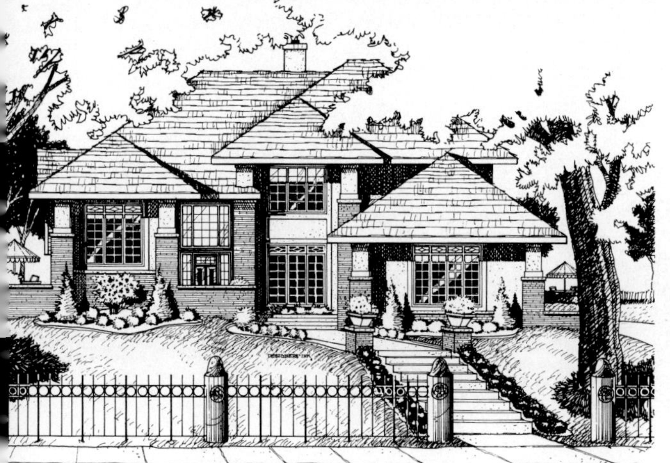

MID-LEVEL GET-AWAY

Main Floor: 1735 Sq. Ft.
Second Floor: 841 Sq. Ft.
Total Square Feet: 2576 Sq. Ft.

Hanna

#28A-4081 Plan Price $585

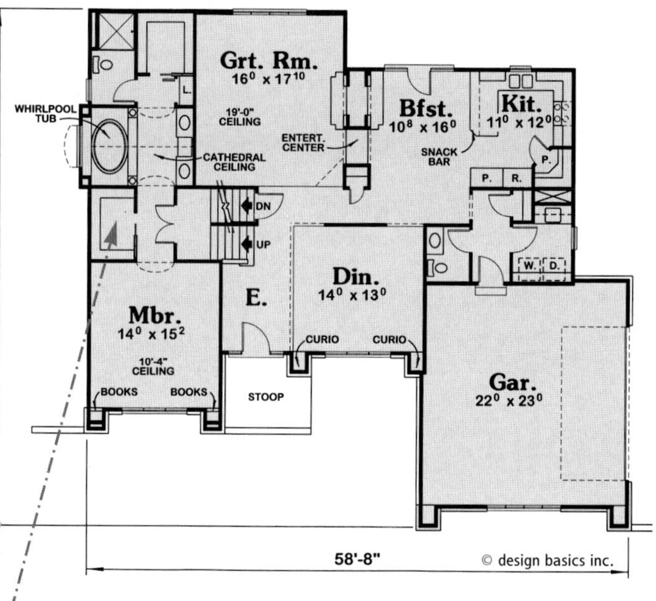

...urious mid-level master suite fea- ...two walk-in closets, built-in book- ...s and a whirlpool tub framed by ...d columns and a cathedral ceiling.

The two-story great room is enjoyed by a view from the second floor corridor.

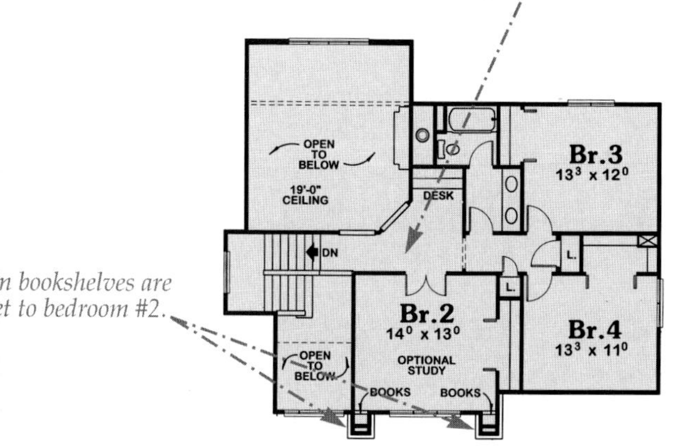

...n bookshelves are ...t to bedroom #2.

SECLUDED IN LUXURY

Main Floor: 1933 Sq. Ft.
Second Floor: 646 Sq. Ft.
Total Square Feet: 2579 Sq. Ft.

Edmonton

#28A-2309 Plan Price $585

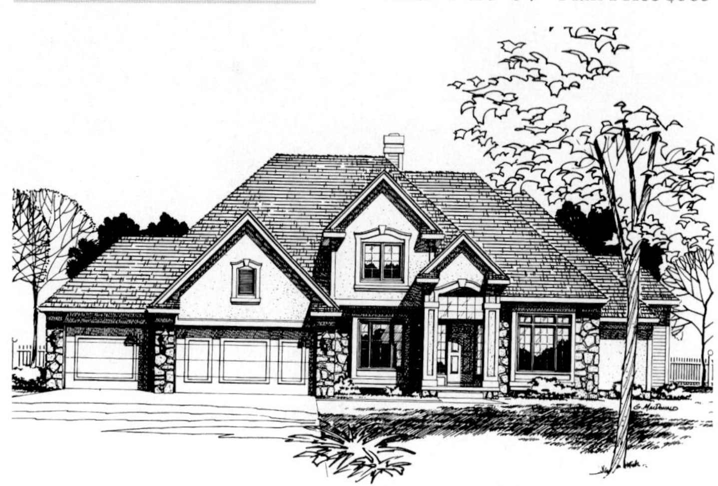

A built-in bookcase enhances the entrance to the master suite, featuring an oval whirlpool tub and volume ceiling.

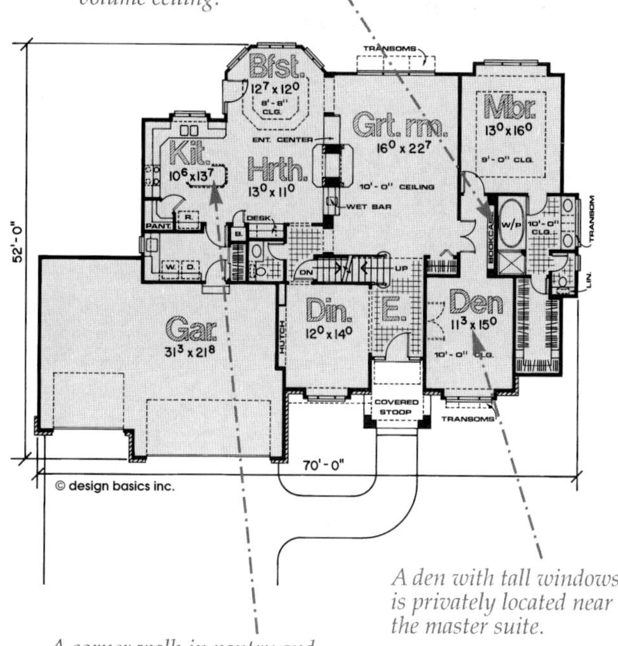

A den with tall windows is privately located near the master suite.

A corner walk-in pantry and island counter benefit the hearth kitchen.

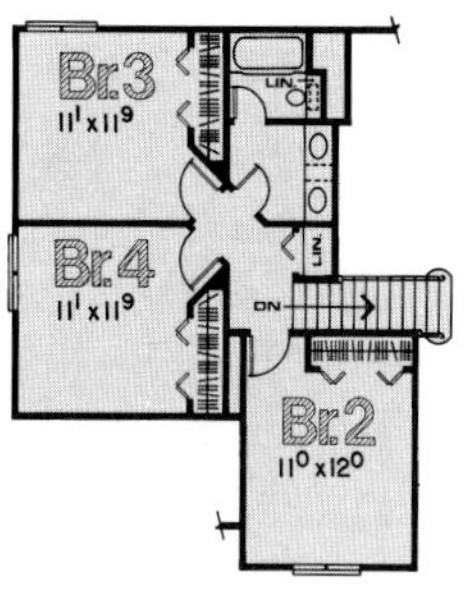

SEPARATE WALK-INS

Main Floor: 2500 Sq. Ft.
Second Floor: 973 Sq. Ft.
Total Square Feet: 3473 Sq. Ft.

Carlton

#28A-1588 Plan Price $675

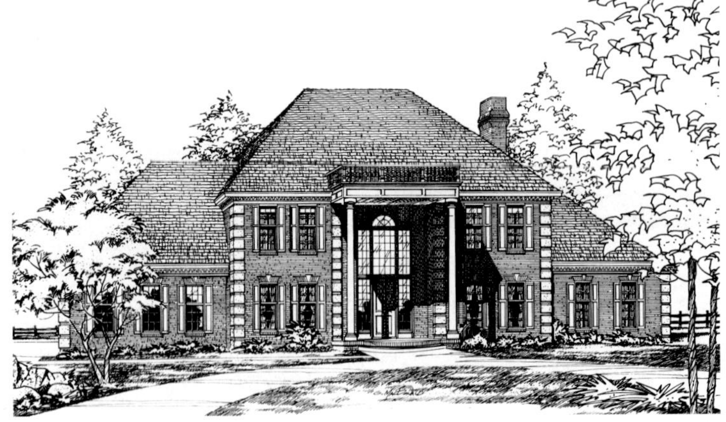

Built-in shelves benefit one of the two large walk-in closets in the master suite.

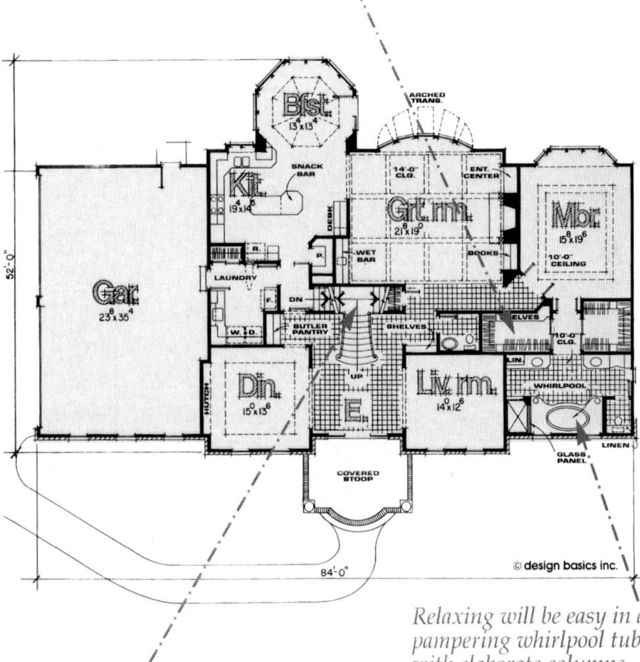

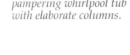

Relaxing will be easy in a pampering whirlpool tub with elaborate columns.

A stunning T-shaped stairway floods the entry, tempting guests to the second floor.

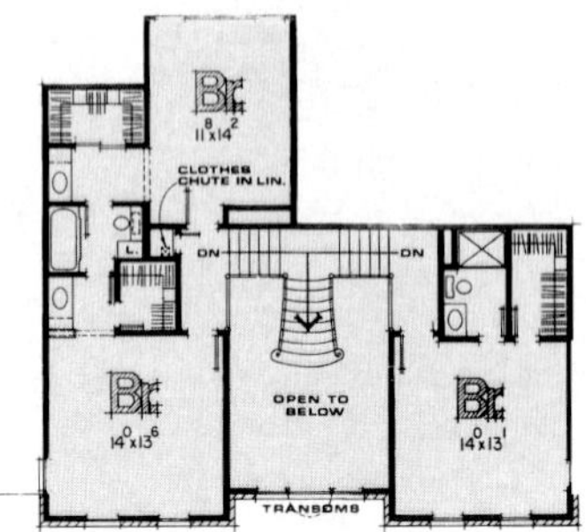

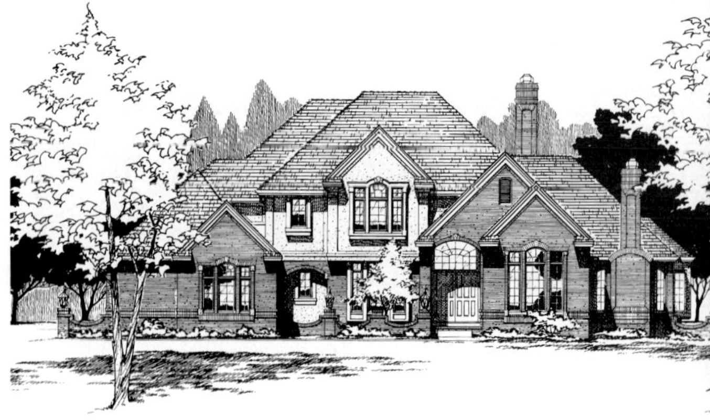

FIRESIDE SITTING ROOM

Main Floor: 2603 Sq. Ft.
Second Floor: 1020 Sq. Ft.
Total Square Feet: 3623 Sq. Ft.

Canterbury

#28A-2411 Plan Price $695

A separate make-up counter across from an extravagant whirlpool tub adds convenience to the master bath.

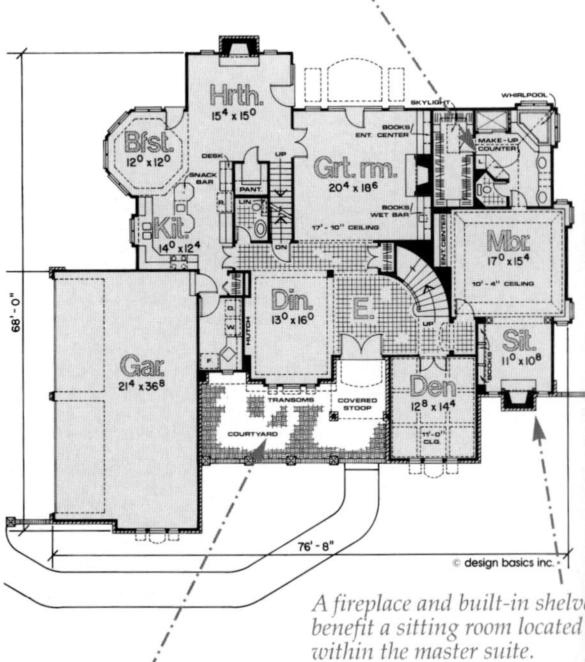

A fireplace and built-in shelves benefit a sitting room located within the master suite.

The front courtyard is a wonderful place to entertain guests or show off greenery.

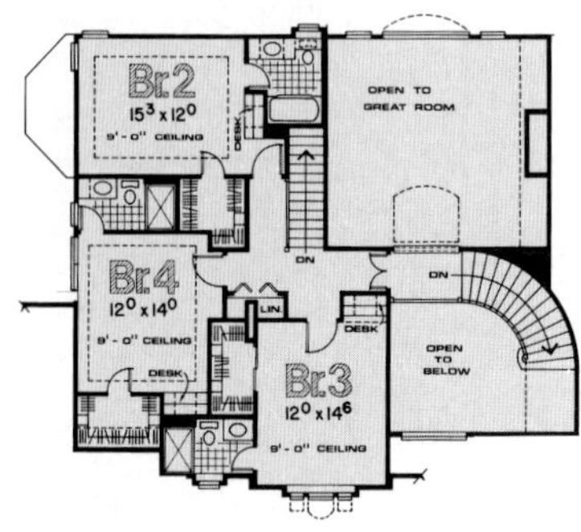

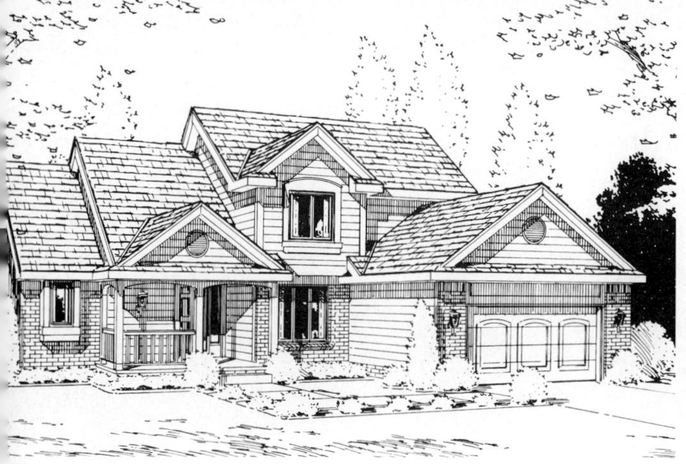

Sunlit corner tub

Main Floor: 1398 Sq. Ft.
Second Floor: 598 Sq. Ft.
Total Square Feet: 1996 Sq. Ft.

Stevens Woods

#28A-8053 Plan Price $425

mong the relaxing amenities in the aster bedroom are a volume ceiling d beautiful views to the back.

A snack bar serves the sunny bayed breakfast area.

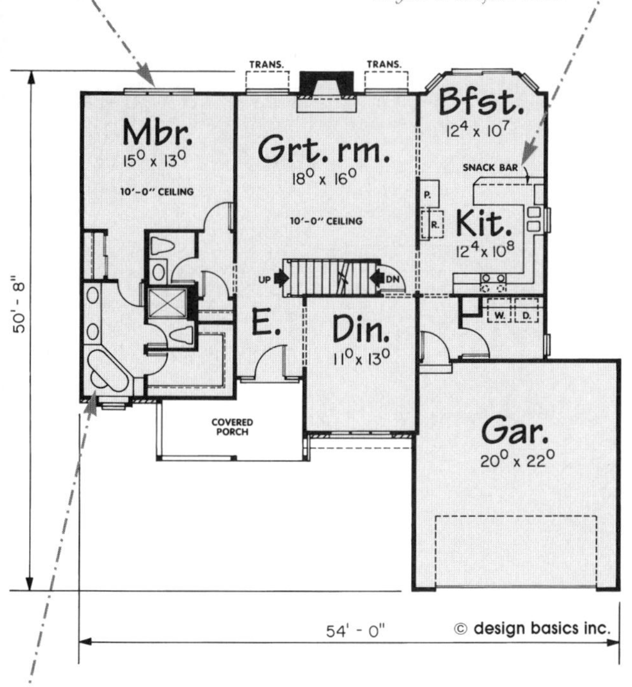

e roomy master bath features a rner soaking tub under glass d a dual-sink vanity.

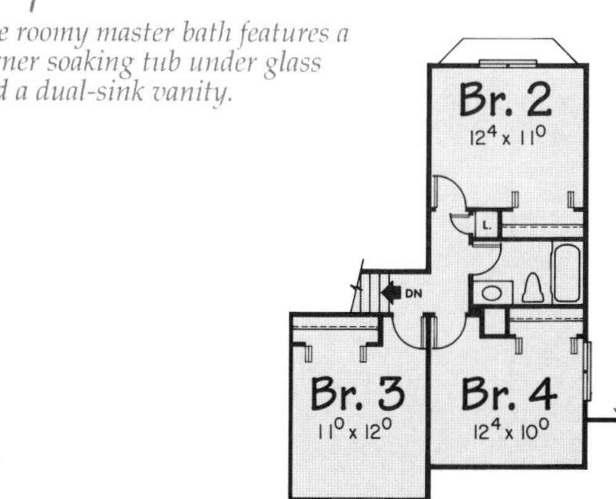

Romantic whirlpool tub

Main Floor: 1551 Sq. Ft.
Second Floor: 725 Sq. Ft.
Total Square Feet: 2276 Sq. Ft.

Chandler

#28A-1554 Plan Price $555

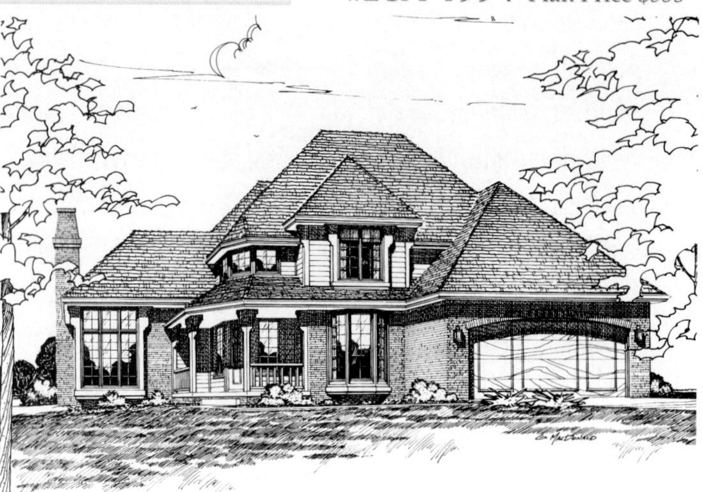

A vaulted ceiling and corner windows add luster to the master bedroom.

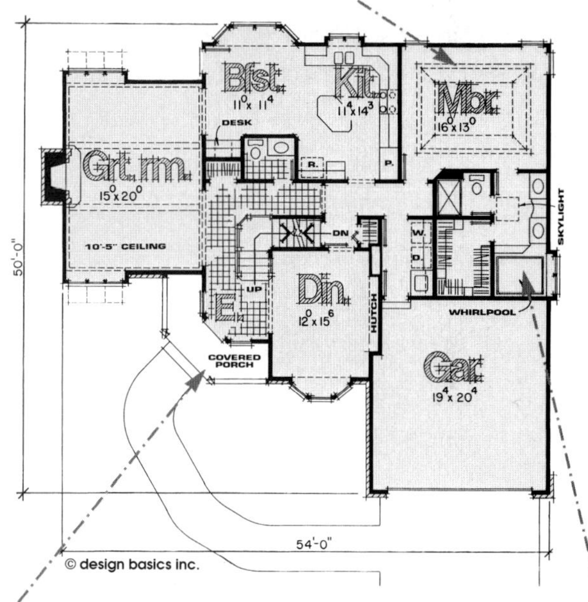

The angle of the front porch adds beauty to the home's exterior curb appeal.

A two-person whirlpool tub and skylit vanity give a romantic air to the master bath.

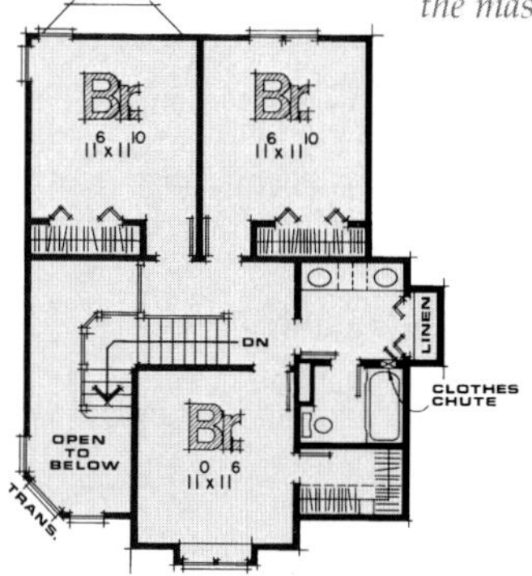

I've always wanted to be a fireman. I'm one of the old-timers who didn't have television growing up, so radio was solace to this adolescent passion. Every Friday night a popular serial about firemen would come on the air and I would relish the stories of the latest death-defying firefighter or heroic animal rescue. I would lie on our living room rug imagining it was me, saving innocent children from the most impossible fires. This is the man I thought I wanted to write about someday. It was only when I got older that I realized I had to climb a 100-foot ladder to become a fireman. I never did try out.

I've always wanted to be a fireman. I'm one of the old-timers who didn't have television growing up, so radio was solace to this adolescent passion.

My real life story is this: I was born in 1934, the youngest of eight children. My father was a butcher who worked for a local meat packing plant in the central part of town. My mother - indicative of the times - stayed home to raise us. I joined the navy when I was 19 years old, catching the tail end of the Korean War. After the navy, I became a police officer and later worked as a security guard, handyman and maintenance man. An ailing back prompted me to retire this year. This is my life in a nutshell.

I find it surprising that, now that I'm retired, people ask me how I've done it - what's kept me going all of these years. It's as though they're looking for the secret of life in the midst of their day-to-day drudgery and somehow think I've found it. I don't know if I have, but what I tell them is that besides my deep faith in God, my home has been a constant source of strength in my life.

There's nothing special about the home I live in now, but I still see the little things about it that said "yes" to us when we first looked at it. We liked the master suite with its private bath. We liked having all the rooms on one floor. We loved its openness in the back and built-in bookshelves in the basement. For me specifically, it was the yard. Both the front and back of the home have wonderful trees, hedges and landscaping. My yard is my hobby - making sure the hedges are clipped, the flowers watered and the lawn mowed. To me my lawn is like freedom. It's a place I can mold into something of beauty and structure. But since I've hurt my back, I'm unable to maintain it without the help of friends. Sitting in this chair "recovering," I miss it more than you can imagine.

Marcell

#28A-4133 Plan Price $505

Main Floor:	1314 Sq. Ft.
Second Floor:	458 Sq. Ft.
Total Square Feet:	1772 Sq. Ft.

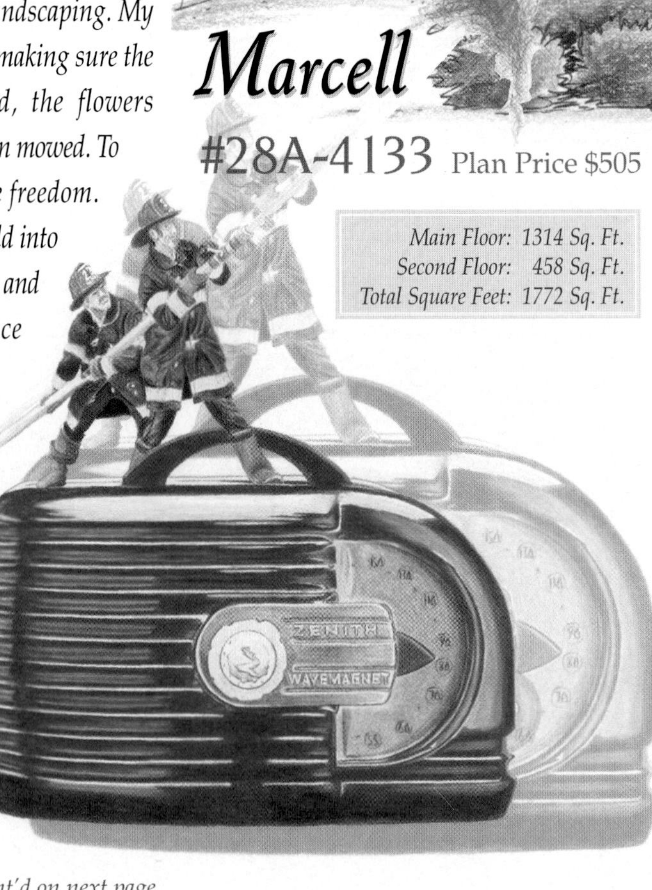

cont'd on next page

design basics inc. HOME PLAN DESIGN SERVICE

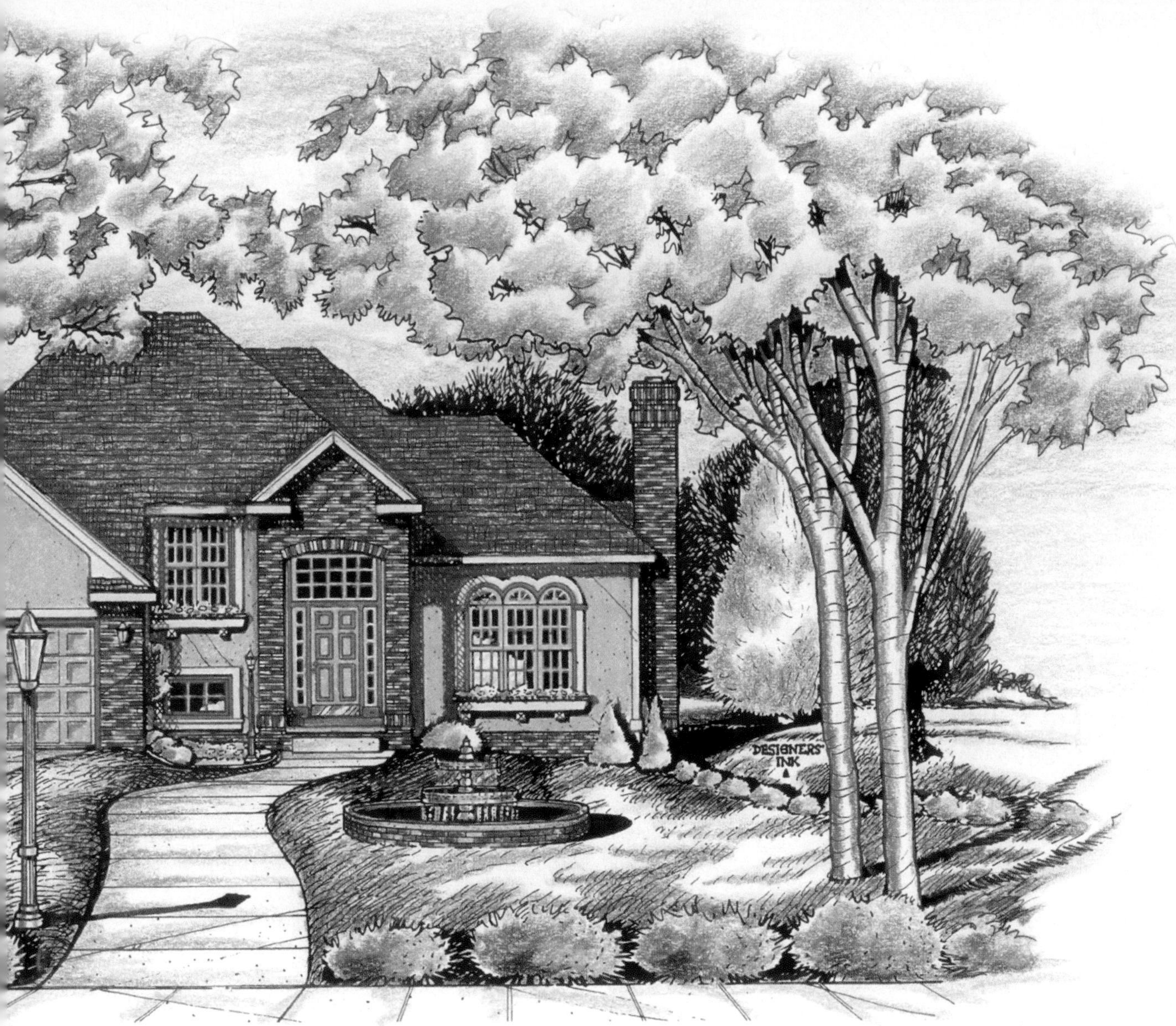

An island counter in the kitchen is within steps of the stove and sink, making it convenient when cooking.

The great room offers views and accessibility from both the front and rear of the home.

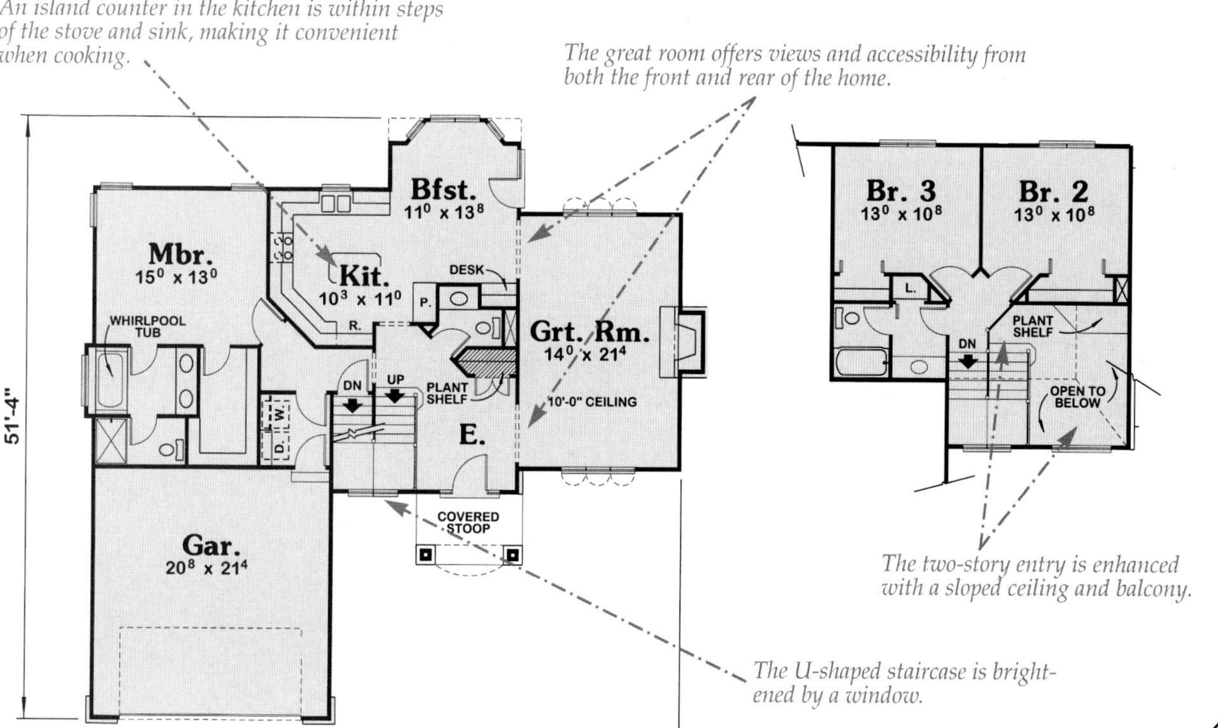

The two-story entry is enhanced with a sloped ceiling and balcony.

The U-shaped staircase is brightened by a window.

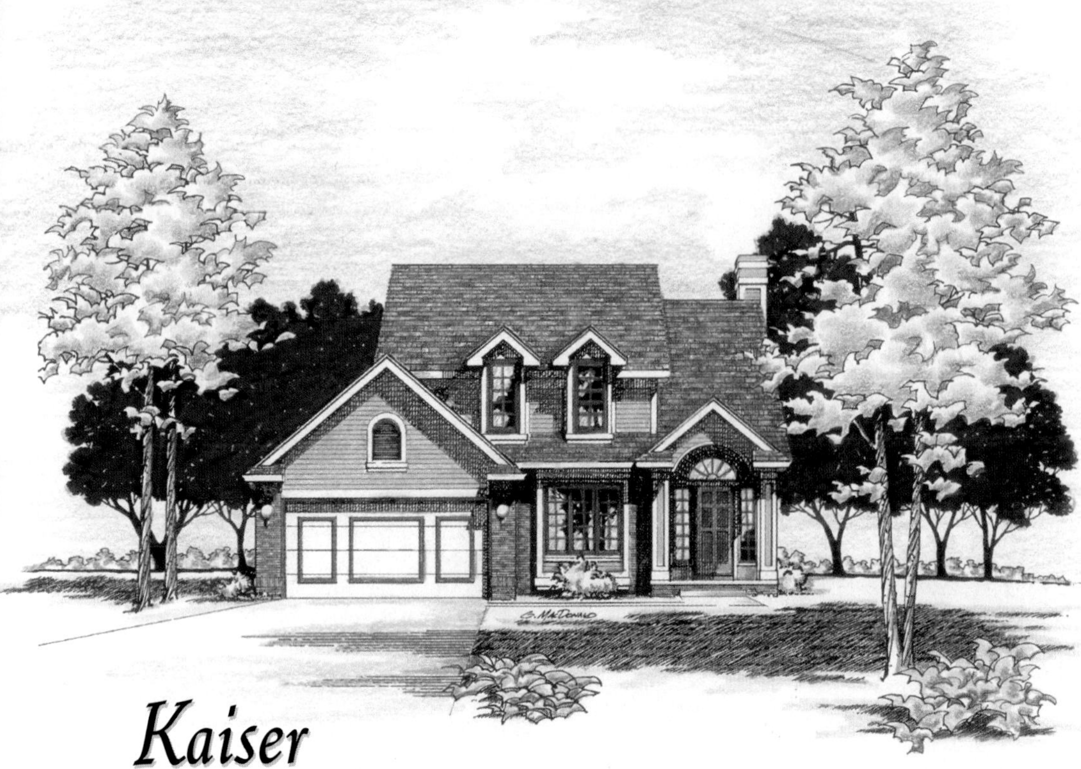

Kaiser

#28A-2578 Plan Price $495

Main Floor:	1327 Sq. Ft.
Second Floor:	348 Sq. Ft.
Total Square Feet:	1675 Sq. Ft.

The master suite is secluded at the rear of the home.

Large windows allow the kitchen/breakfast area to be flooded with natural light.

TRANSOMS
Mbr. 14⁰ x 13⁰ 9'-0" CEILING
Bfst. 11⁴ x 10⁰ 10'-0" CEILING
SNACK BAR
Kit. 11⁴ x 9⁰
Grt. rm. 14⁰ x 18⁶ 10'-8" CEILING
WHIRL-POOL
LIN.
W.
D.
DN
UP
E.
Din. 11⁰ x 14⁰
Gar. 19⁴ x 22⁰
COVERED STOOP
53' - 0"
40' - 8"
© design basics inc.

A high ceiling and expansive views through the great room's tall windows provide powerful first impressions upon entering the home.

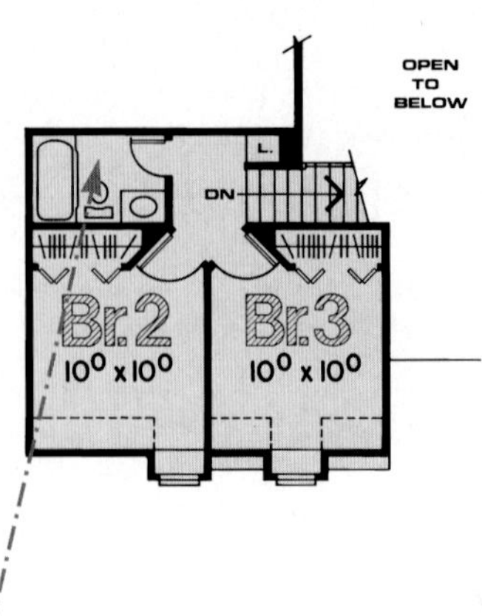

Upstairs bedrooms share a convenient hall bath and two linen closets.

My yard is my hobby – making sure the hedges are clipped, the flowers watered and the lawn mowed. To me my lawn is like freedom.

Many of my friends have cabins or other places they "get away to" on the weekends. My home has been the place I get away to. It's helped create th memories I've enjoyed returning t over the years. I think of a home as place that's the center of my family. have two wonderful daughters, bot single. Their mother has passe away and I've since remarried. On lives near me and the other is in Sa Diego. But no matter where the are, my house will always b "home" to them.

It's not as though I have an special attachment to this particu lar place. My family and I hav lived in a lot of houses, but "home has always come along with u Home is much more than whe I've hung my hat - it's like the oth saying - it's where my heart has been.

cont'd on next page

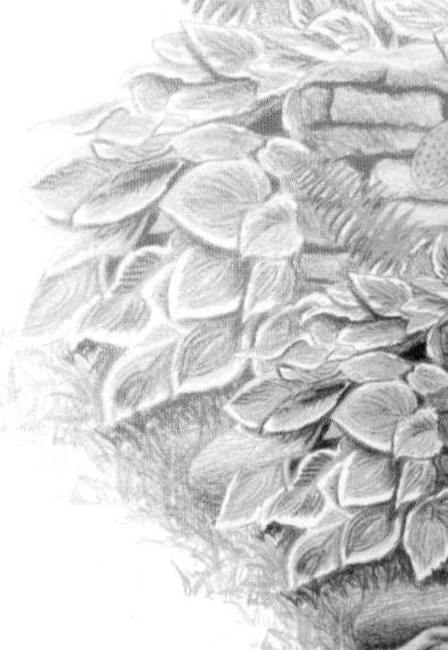

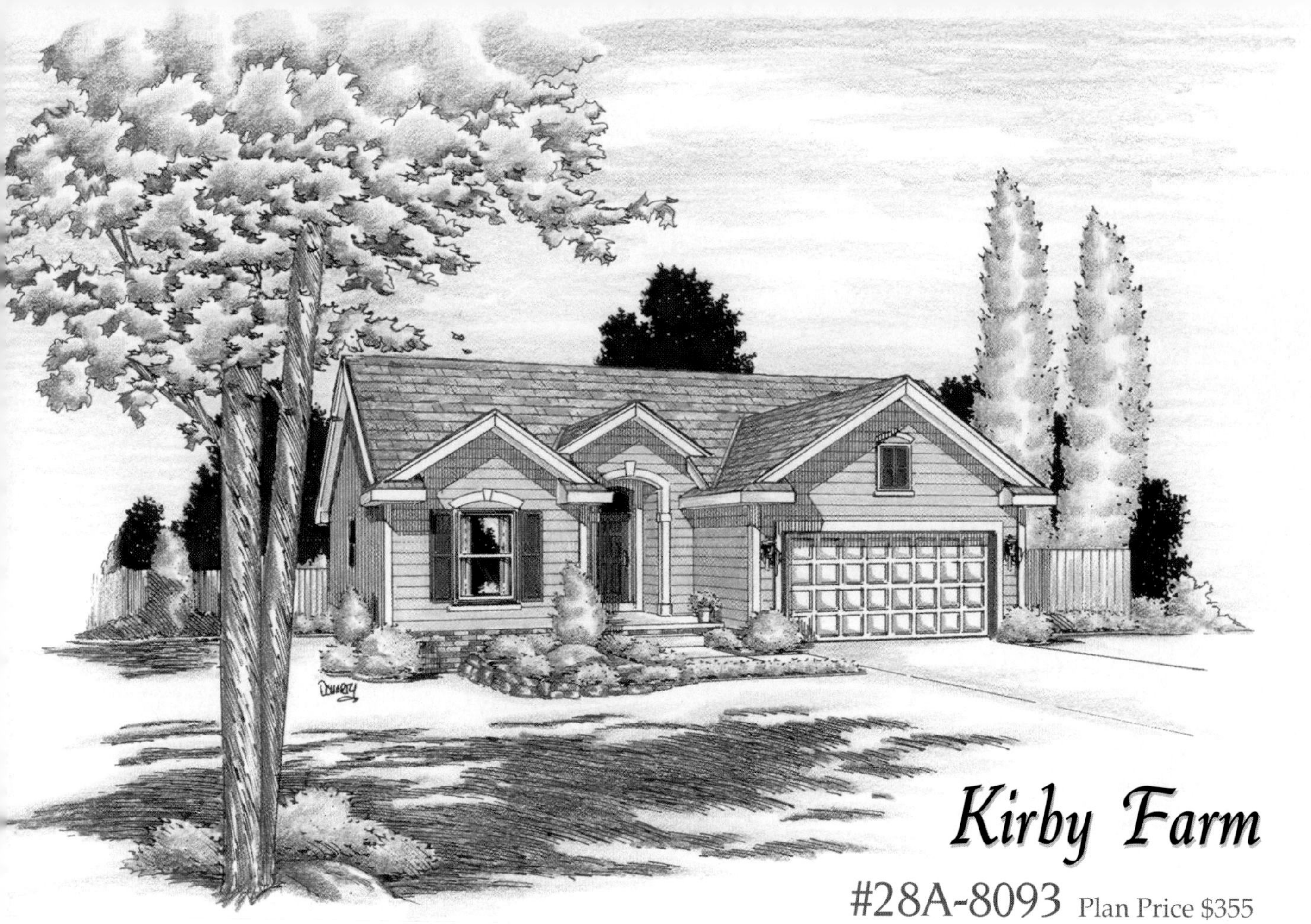

Kirby Farm

#28A-8093 Plan Price $355

Total Square Feet: 1212 Sq. Ft.

The master suite is situated for privacy at the rear of the home.

The second bedroom easily converts into a private study or home office.

The kitchen/breakfast area is well planned with plenty of counter space and a built-in snack bar.

For cozy nights near the fireplace, the great room offers a built-in bookcase.

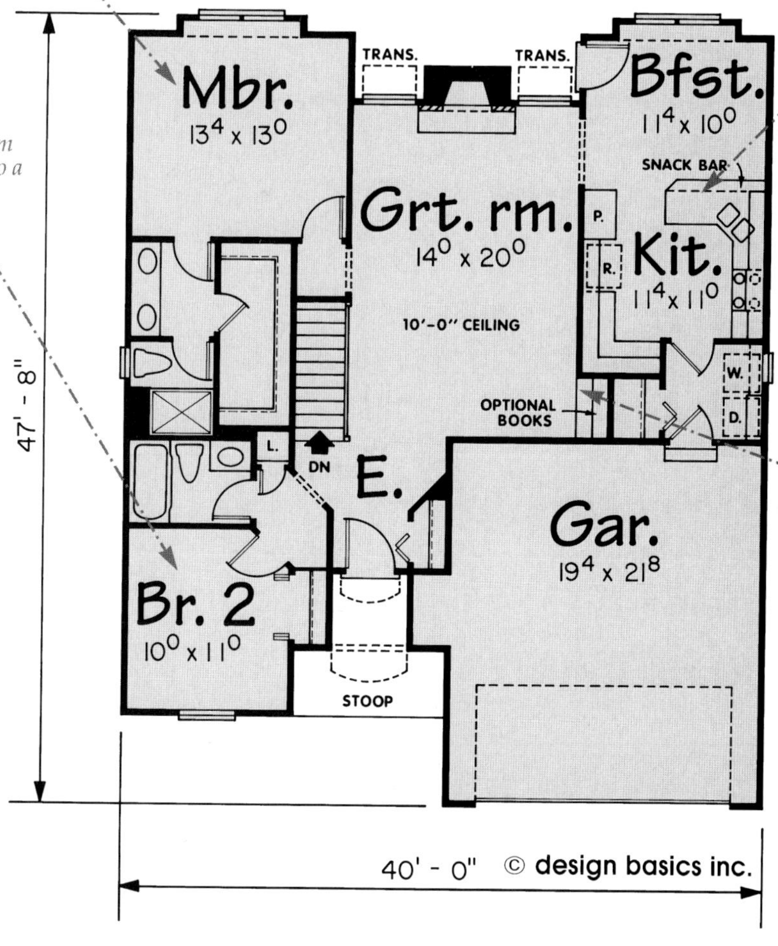

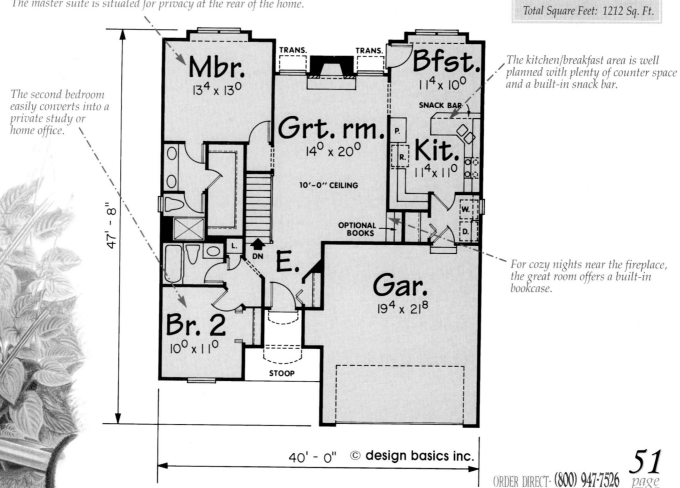

© design basics inc.

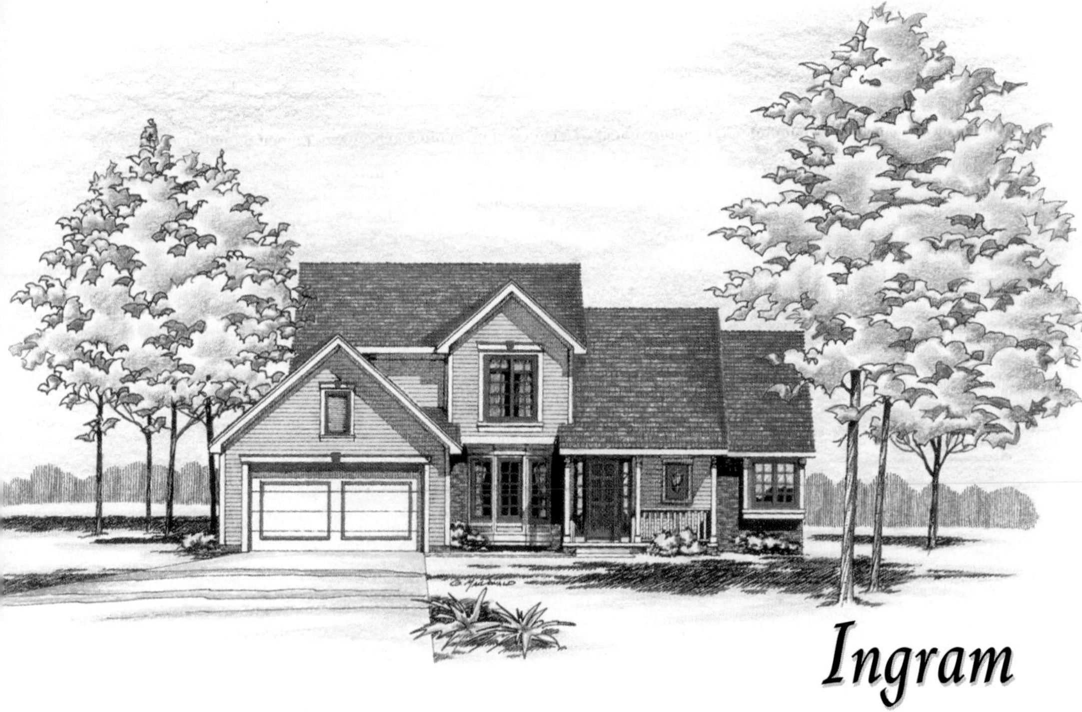

Ingram

#28A-2281 Plan Price $505

Main Floor: 1348 Sq. Ft.
Second Floor: 430 Sq. Ft.
Total Square Feet: 1778 Sq. Ft.

LIN.
DN
Br.3 12⁴x10¹
Br.2 12⁰x11³

The great room enhances any gathering with its high, sloped ceiling and fireplace flanked by windows.

The master suite provides a sense of luxury with its special ceiling details and pampering bath area.

Bfst. 12⁴x10⁸
SNACK BAR
Kit. 12⁴x10⁸
P.
R.
Grt. rm. 18⁰x16⁰
SLOPED CEILING
Mbr. 15⁰x13⁰
10'-0" CLG.
DN
UP
E.
W.
D.
SHELVES
HUTCH
Din. 12⁰x13⁰
W/P
COVERED PORCH
Gar. 20⁷x24⁷
48'-8"
54'-0"

© design basics inc.

Extra space in the garage includes the convenience of built-in shelves.

Meals are prepared just steps away from the formal bayed dining room.

So many of my days are now spent visiting over coffee in the afternoon with friends and family who live nearby.

When I think of home in this way, I can only recall one time in which a sense of home did not come with me and that was the time I spent in the navy. There, home was a place I longed to come back to. Out on the sea, deep in the ship's hull, it was what I lived for until my years of service were up.

I think of how we've lived in our home. The previous owner rarely used the main floor, spending most of their time in the family room of the basement. Not us. Our living room is where we watch our sitcoms and home improvement shows on the weekends. When we moved in the dining room carpet was white. It's now visibly dulled from use.

This concept of home also makes me think of my daily life. So many of my days are now spent visiting over coffee in the afternoon with friends and family who live nearby. Our conversations weave a trail unnoticed, all along the way, home growing deeper into ourselves with each story about a neighbor or politician or doctor visit.

It also makes me think of our book-

cont'd on next page

design basics inc. HOME PLAN DESIGN SERVICE

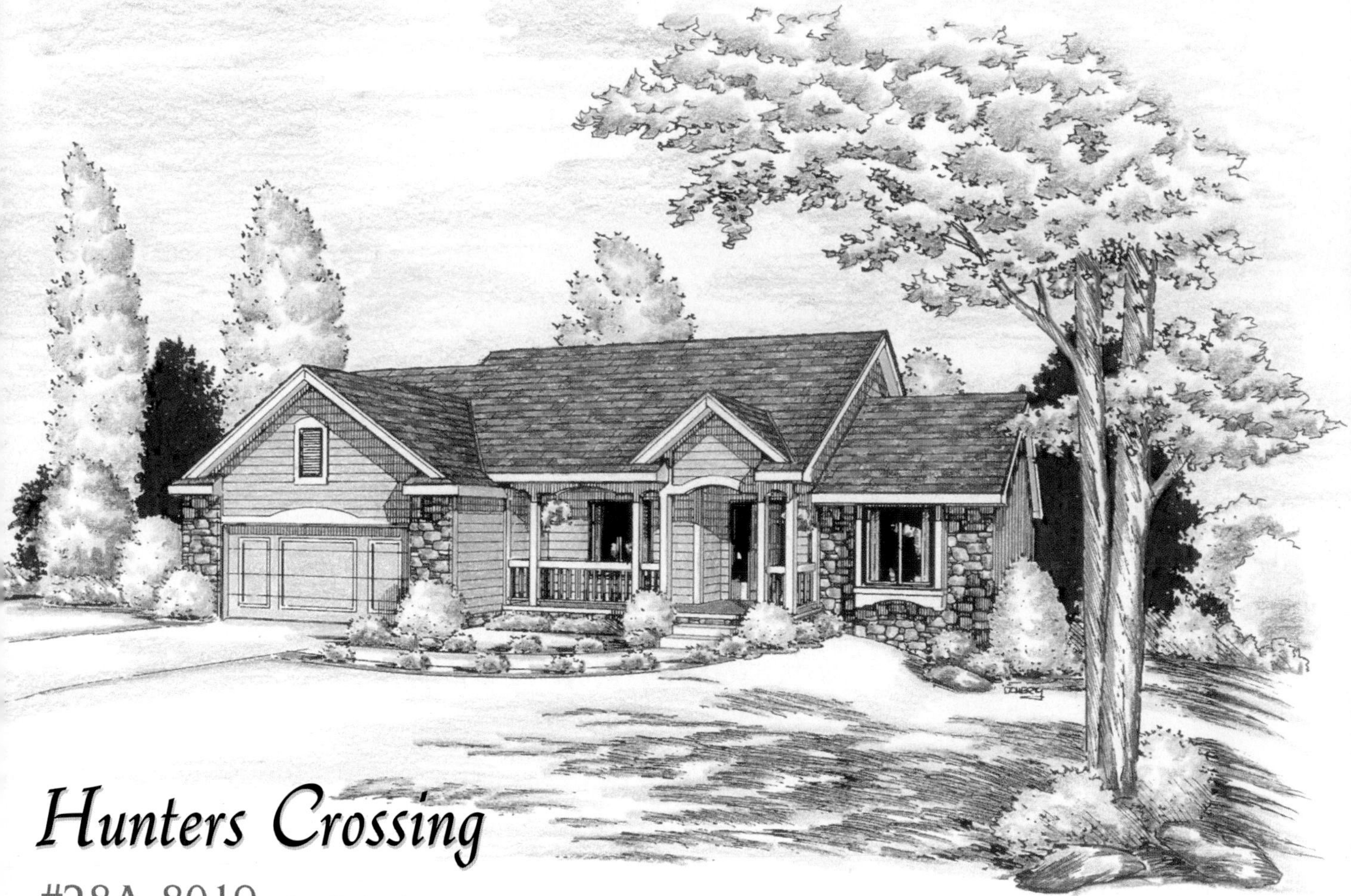

Hunters Crossing

#28A-8019 Plan Price $425

Total Square Feet: 1919 Sq. Ft.

Openness between the kitchen, breakfast area and hearth room make this area a natural place for daily living.

Secluded from the master suite, the secondary bedrooms are perfect for guests or a live-in parent.

The master suite features a large vanity to conveniently get ready and an individual soaking tub.

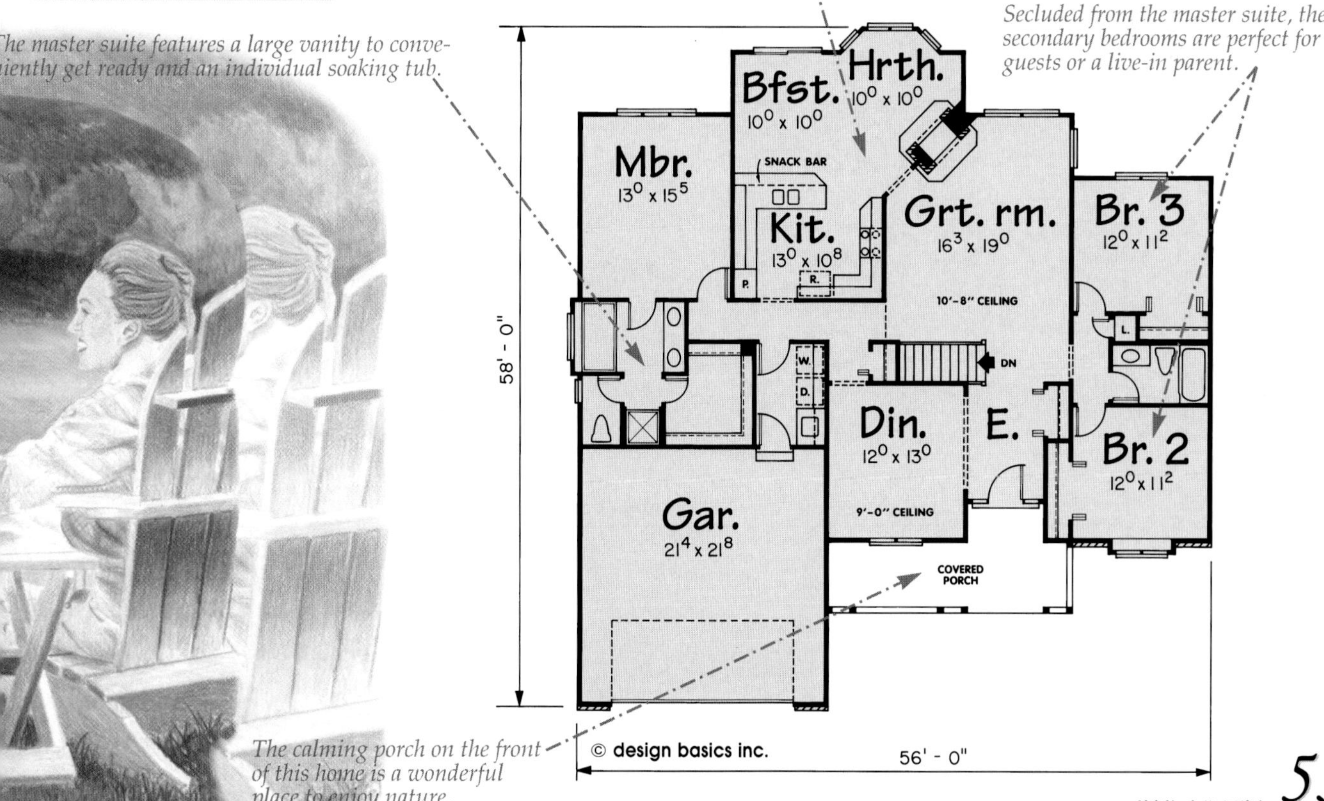

© design basics inc.

The calming porch on the front of this home is a wonderful place to enjoy nature.

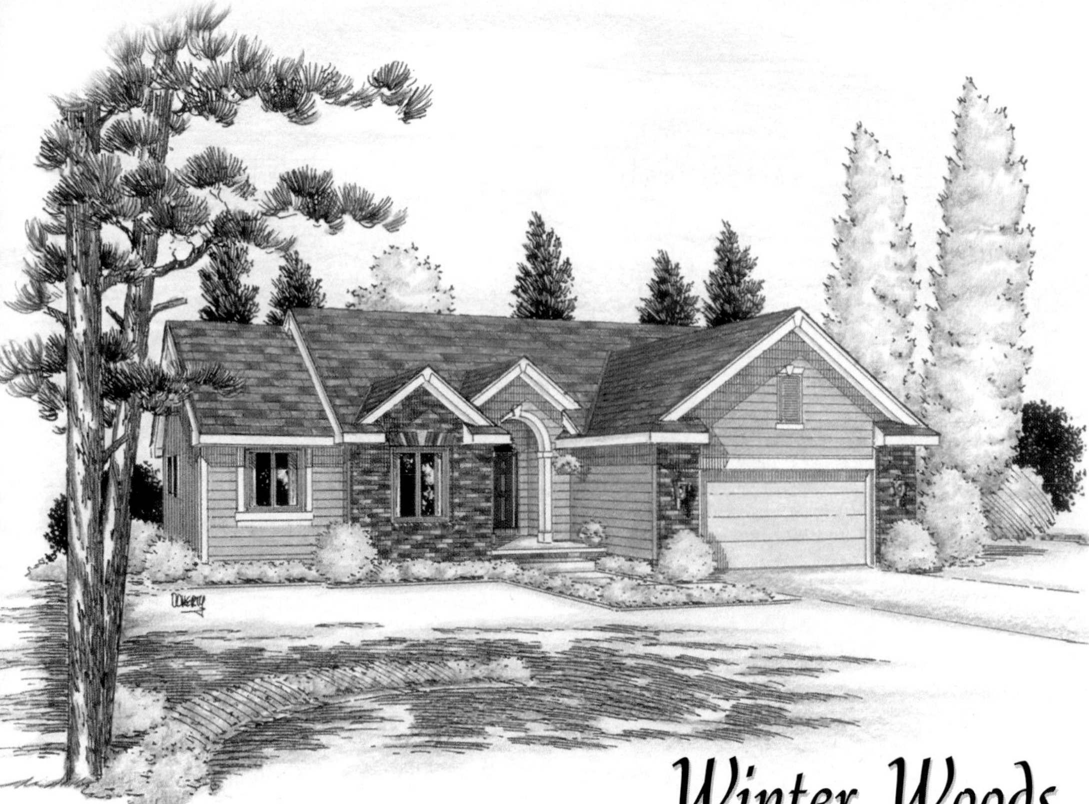

Winter Woods

#28A-8091 Plan Price $365

Total Square Feet: 1360 Sq. Ft.

Upon entering, attention is focused on the airy great room's fireplace, flanked by tall windows.

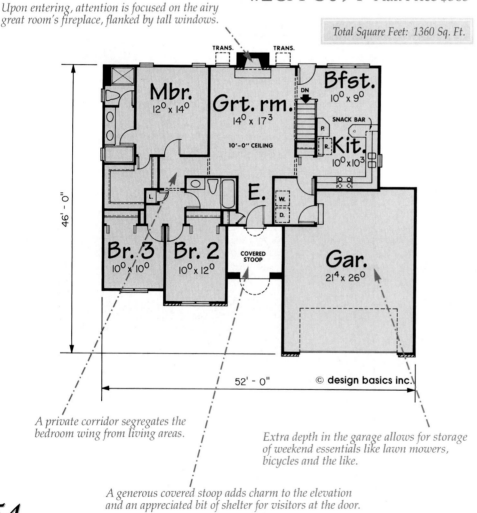

TRANS. TRANS.

Mbr. $12^0 \times 14^0$

Grt. rm. $14^0 \times 17^3$

10'-0" CEILING

Bfst. $10^0 \times 9^0$

DN

SNACK BAR

P. R.

Kit. $10^0 \times 10^3$

L.

E.

W. D.

Br. 3 $10^0 \times 10^0$

Br. 2 $10^0 \times 12^0$

COVERED STOOP

Gar. $21^4 \times 26^0$

46' - 0"

52' - 0"

© design basics inc.

A private corridor segregates the bedroom wing from living areas.

Extra depth in the garage allows for storage of weekend essentials like lawn mowers, bicycles and the like.

A generous covered stoop adds charm to the elevation and an appreciated bit of shelter for visitors at the door.

Her books tend to follow her throughout the house, leaving a trail from coffee table to bed to kitchen counter.

shelves crammed with my wife's mystery and science fiction novels. I think of her extensive collection of cookbooks and how I tease her on the nights we have Hamburger Helper. Her books tend to follow her throughout the house, leaving a trail from coffee table to bed to kitchen counter. I think of my wife reading - curled up in the corner of the couch - her index finger and thumb supporting her head of short red hair. No movement, no sound but the turning of the page.

I think of the comfort of recently returning from the hospital after back surgery, coming home to what's familiar. To our same kitchen. To our worn plaid-patterned couch and the trail of books.

I think of how we probably need a smaller place, where the laundry room is on the main floor. I think of how I probably need fewer rooms to take care of and, for practical reasons, a smaller yard. I think of how I'll soon be ready to move down, bundle up my home and take it with me again. ◆

design basics inc HOME PLAN DESIGN SERVICE

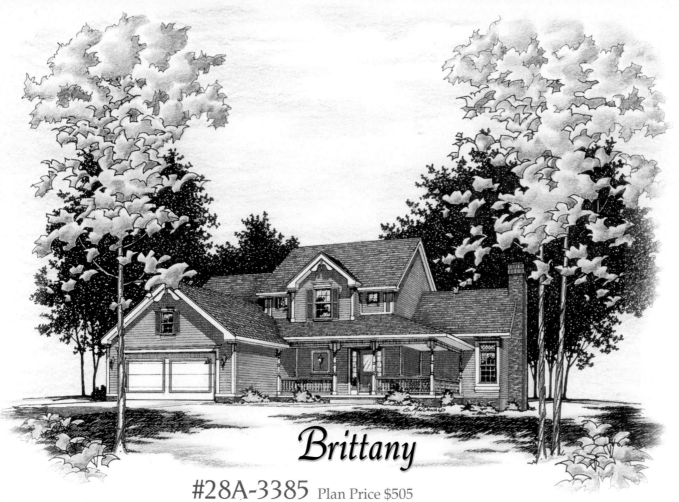

Brittany

#28A-3385 Plan Price $505

Main Floor: 1191 Sq. Ft.
Second Floor: 597 Sq. Ft.
Total Square Feet: 1788 Sq. Ft.

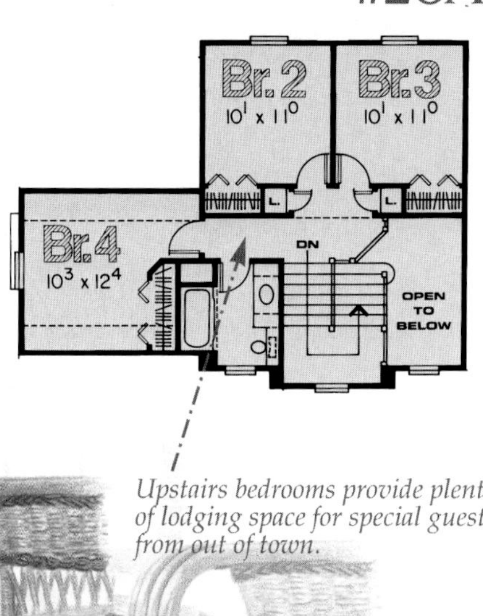

Upstairs bedrooms provide plenty of lodging space for special guests from out of town.

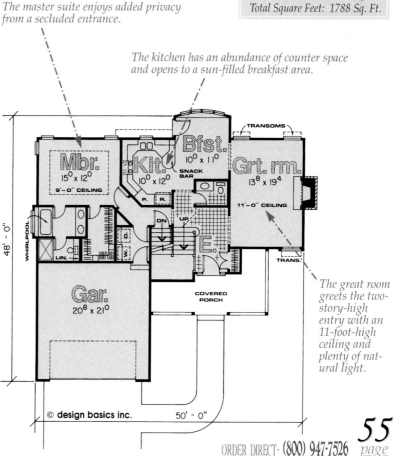

The master suite enjoys added privacy from a secluded entrance.

The kitchen has an abundance of counter space and opens to a sun-filled breakfast area.

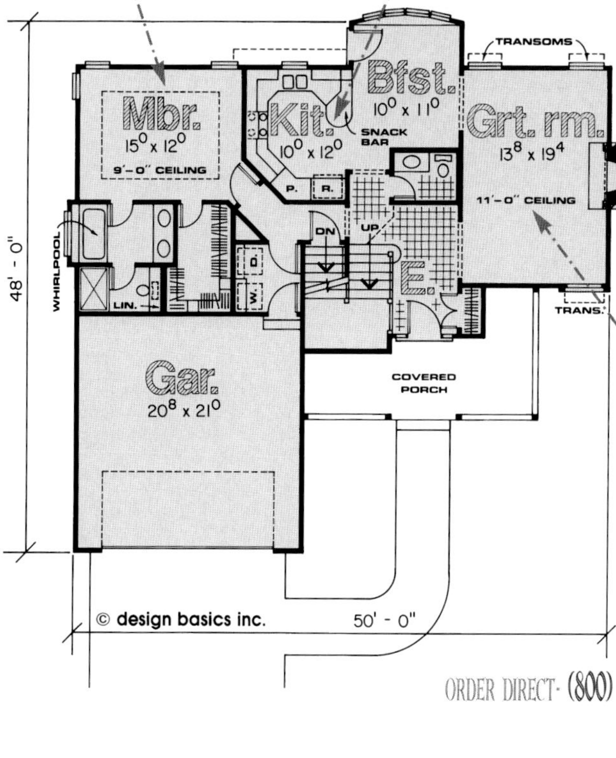

The great room greets the two-story-high entry with an 11-foot-high ceiling and plenty of natural light.

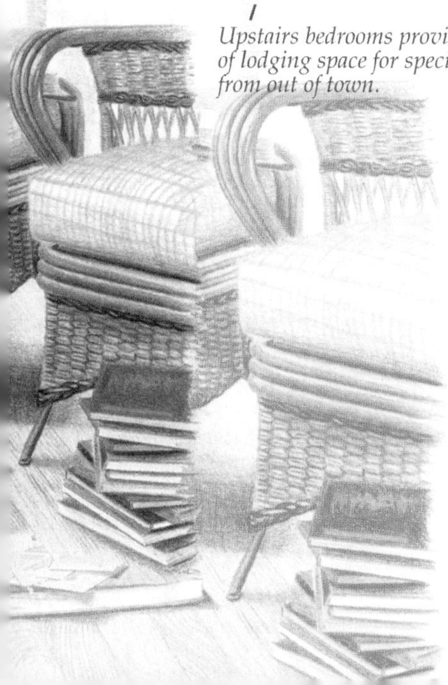

© design basics inc.

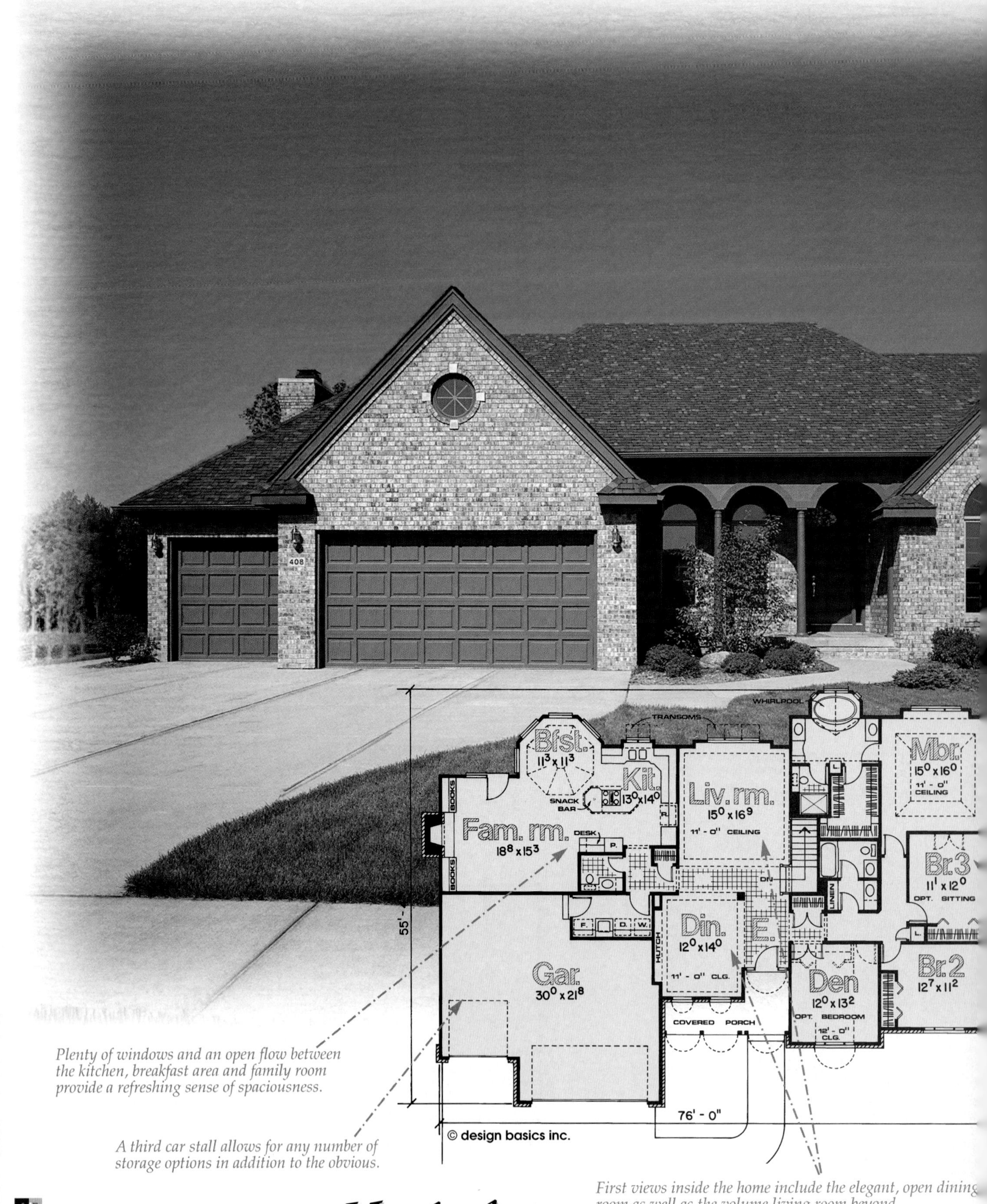

Plenty of windows and an open flow between the kitchen, breakfast area and family room provide a refreshing sense of spaciousness.

A third car stall allows for any number of storage options in addition to the obvious.

First views inside the home include the elegant, open dining room as well as the volume living room beyond.

Hawkesbury

#28A-2206 Plan Price $575

Total Square Feet: 2498 Sq. Ft.

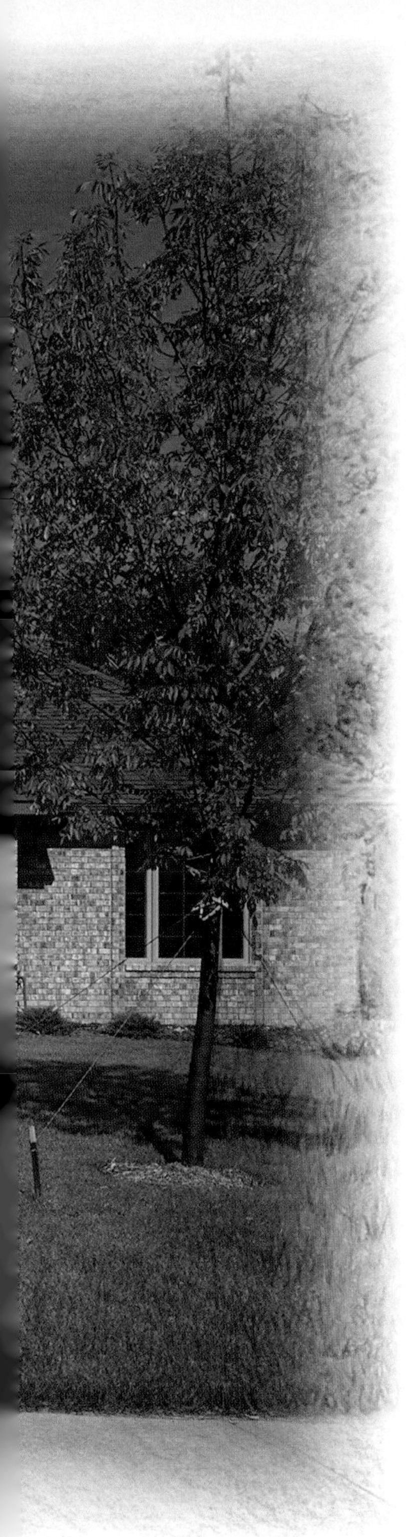

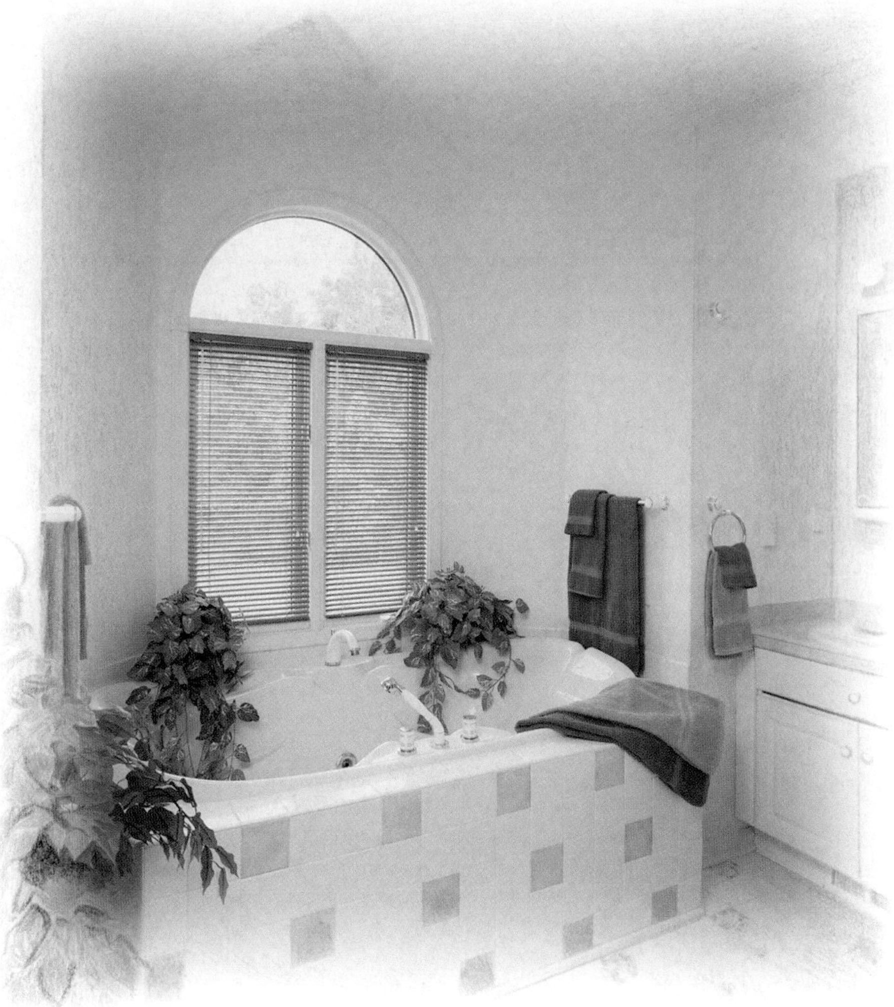

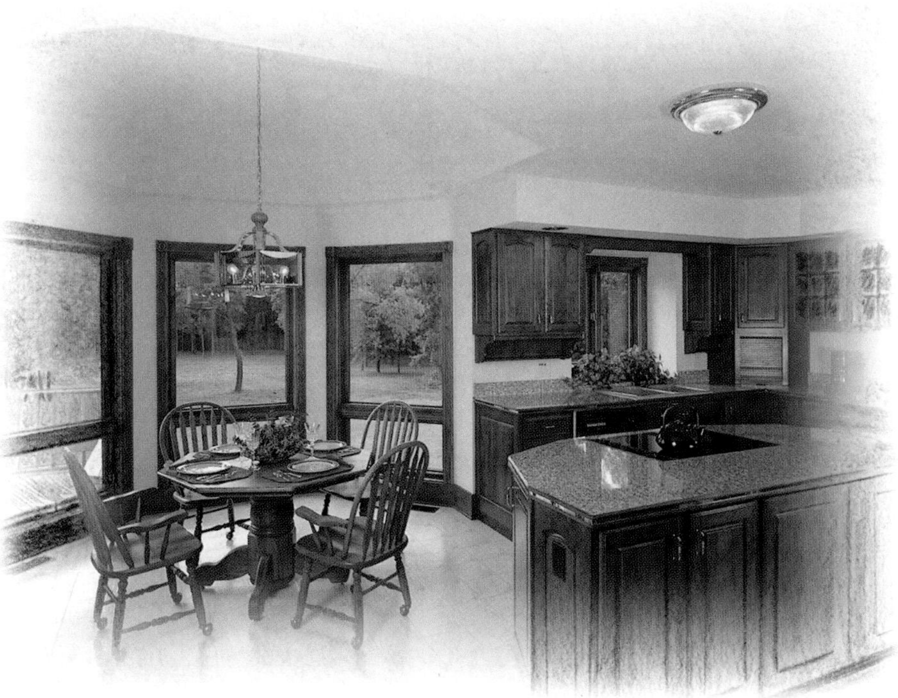

The already generous master suite can be further enlarged by converting the third bedroom into a sitting room.

ABOVE RIGHT: The whirlpool tub in the master suite is flooded with light from an arched window.

BELOW RIGHT: The kitchen inside the Hawkesbury welcomes light from the bayed breakfast area.

ilt By: **Grove Builders Inc.**
Photo By: **Brad Granzow**

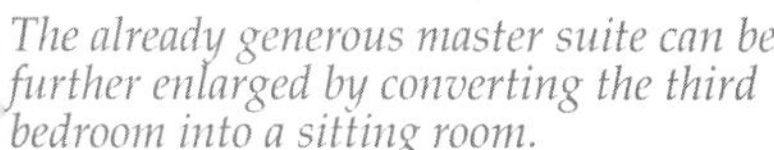

he home in these photographs may be altered from the original plan.

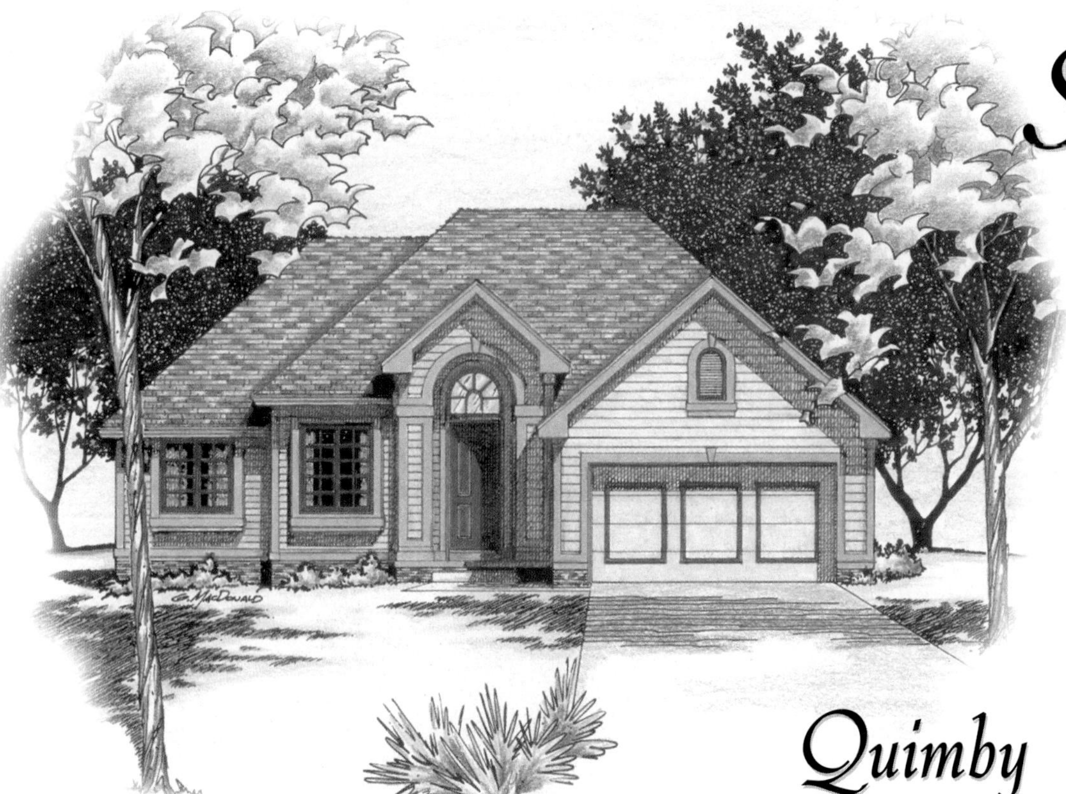

Quimby

#28A-3010 Plan Price $475

SITUATION

I enjoy relaxing after work in my favorite arm chair where I read the paper or watch the news. And after dinner when the dishes are done, I like a place where I can read my favorite magazines and books. I don't need a lot of room – large areas tend to swallow a person up, I think – just a quiet area with a comfortable atmosphere where I can unwind at any time of the day. . .

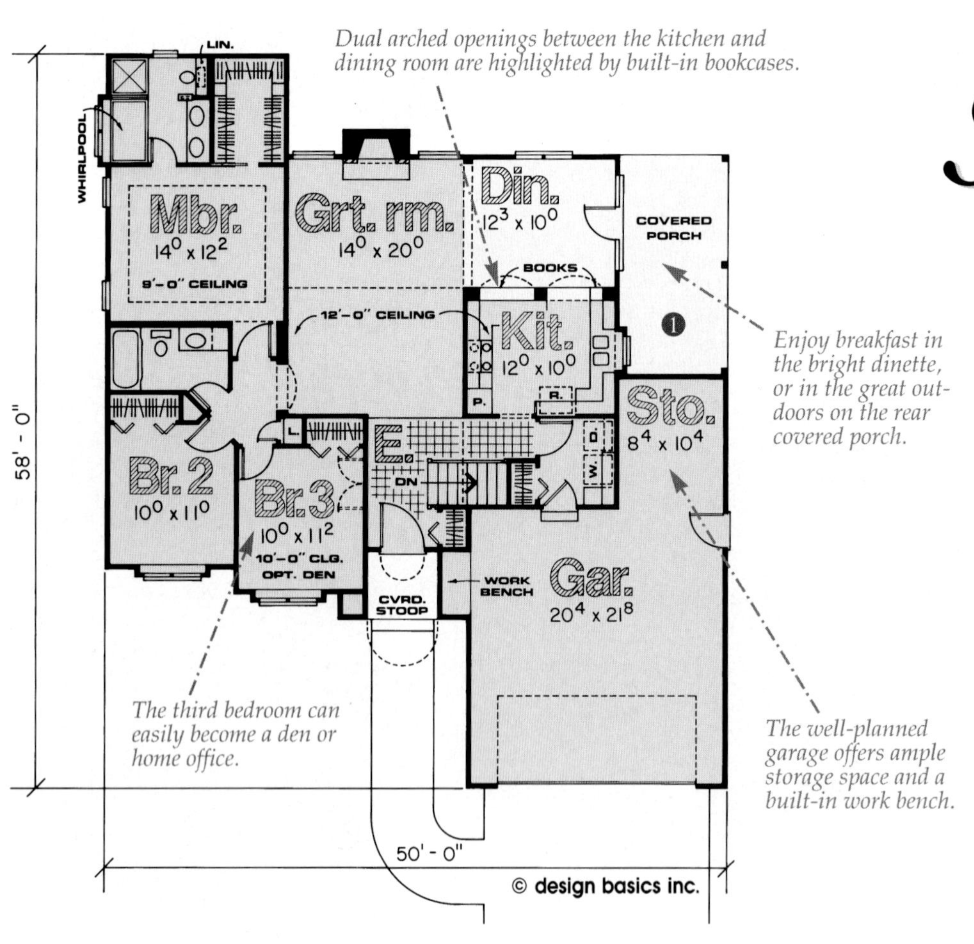

Dual arched openings between the kitchen and dining room are highlighted by built-in bookcases.

Enjoy breakfast in the bright dinette, or in the great outdoors on the rear covered porch.

The third bedroom can easily become a den or home office.

The well-planned garage offers ample storage space and a built-in work bench.

Total Square Feet: 1422 Sq. Ft.

SOLUTION

Both the Lawrence and the Quimby offer wonderful conversation places. The hearth room in the Lawrence (❷, at right and interior view), has a relaxing see-through fireplace, built-in entertainment center and bookshelf. The Quimby's built-in bookshelves are also convenient when you wish to relax with a book either on the covered back porch or in the sun-filled dining room (❶, at left).

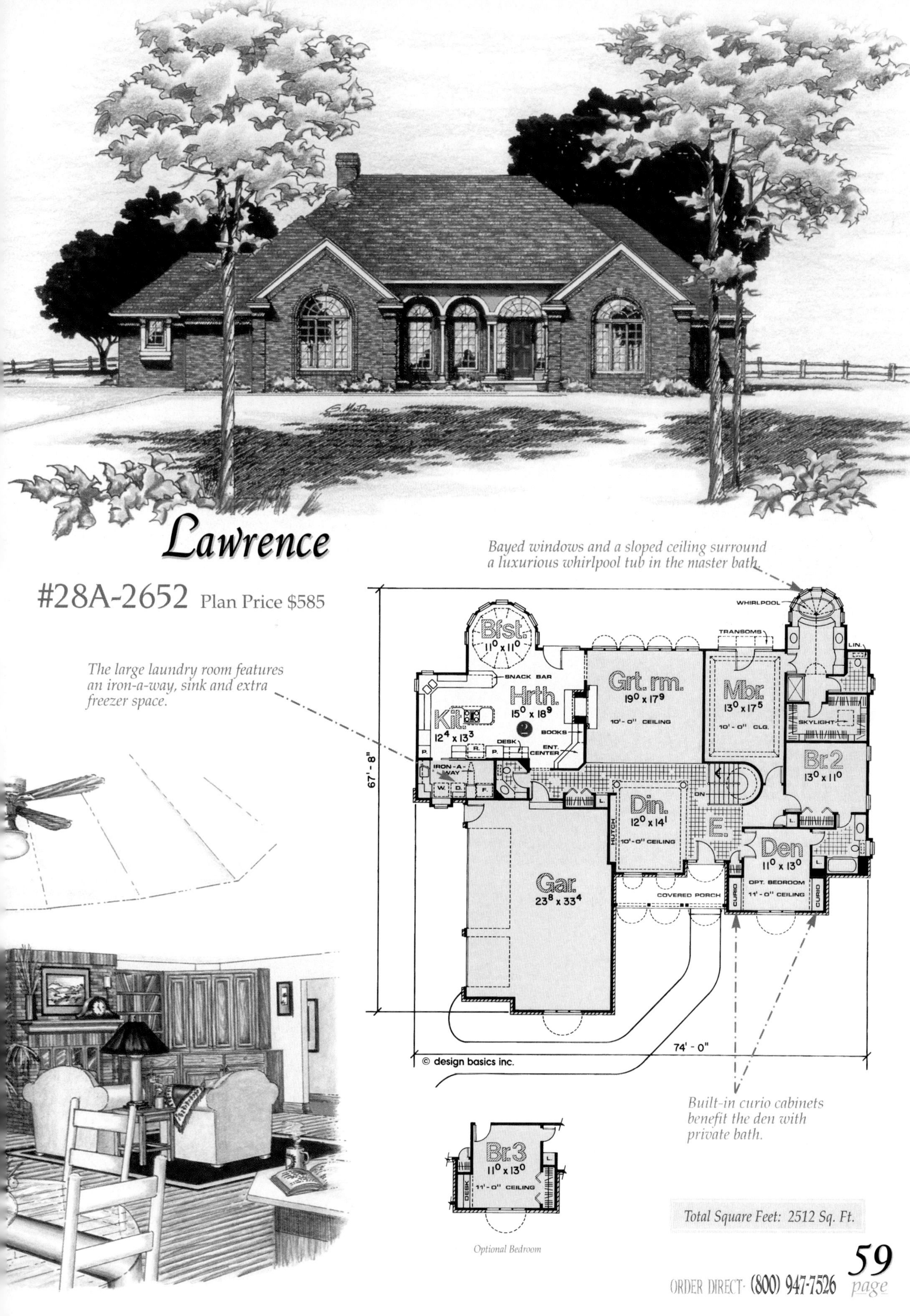

Lawrence

#28A-2652 Plan Price $585

Bayed windows and a sloped ceiling surround a luxurious whirlpool tub in the master bath.

The large laundry room features an iron-a-way, sink and extra freezer space.

Built-in curio cabinets benefit the den with private bath.

Optional Bedroom

Total Square Feet: 2512 Sq. Ft.

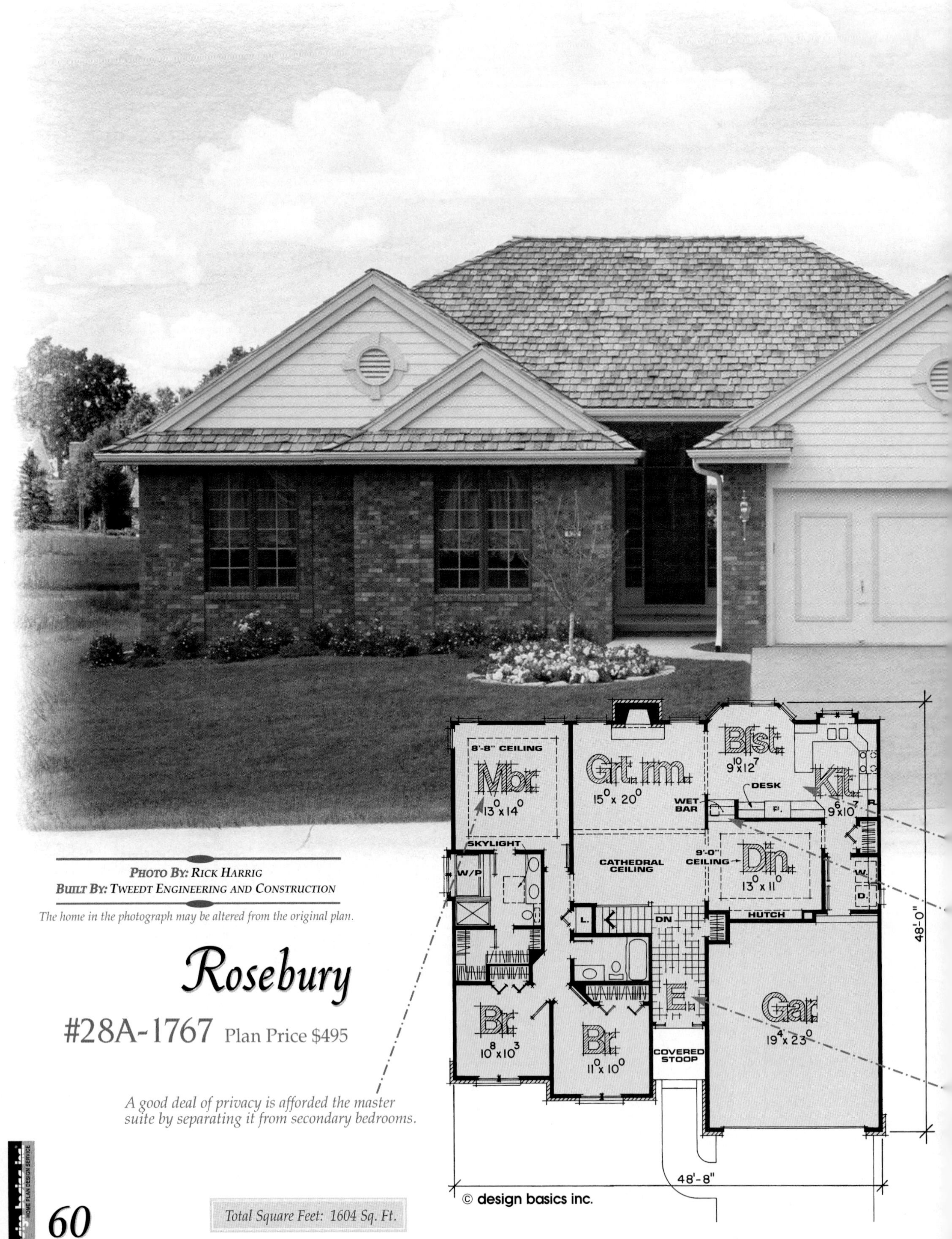

PHOTO BY: RICK HARRIG
BUILT BY: TWEEDT ENGINEERING AND CONSTRUCTION

The home in the photograph may be altered from the original plan.

Rosebury

#28A-1767 Plan Price $495

A good deal of privacy is afforded the master suite by separating it from secondary bedrooms.

Total Square Feet: 1604 Sq. Ft.

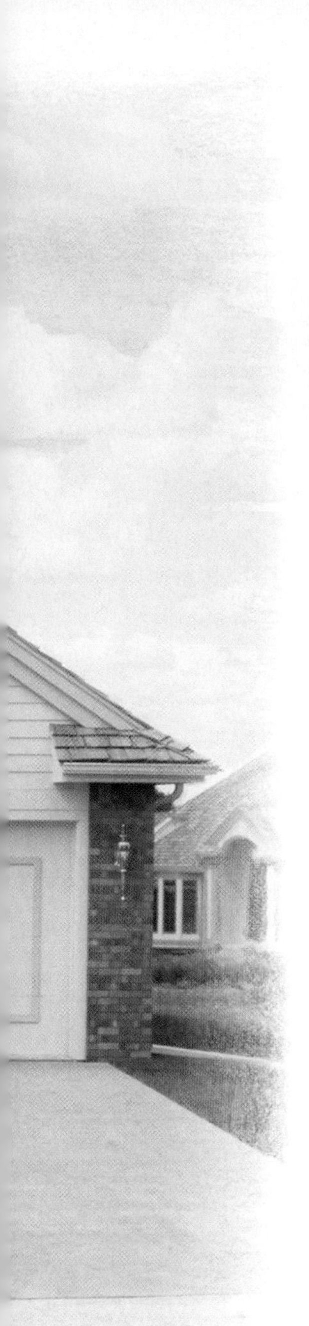

The kitchen enjoys a sense of openness with expansive views into the great room.

A see-thru wet bar conveniently erves both the dining room and reakfast area.

Views from the hard surface entry focus on the great room's fireplace and open vistas beyond.

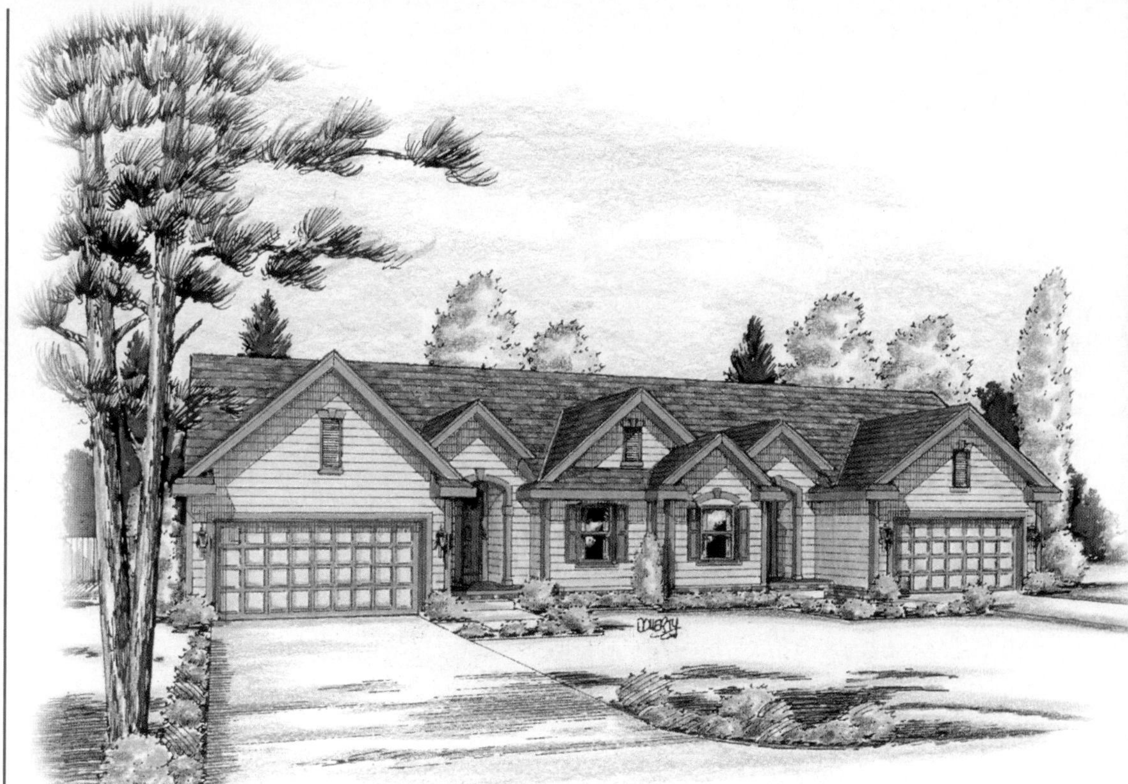

The great room with its fireplace, tall windows and built-in bookcase offers spacious surroundings for a gathering of almost any size.

Master suite's bath area features dual lavs, a walk-in closet and a compartmented stool and shower.

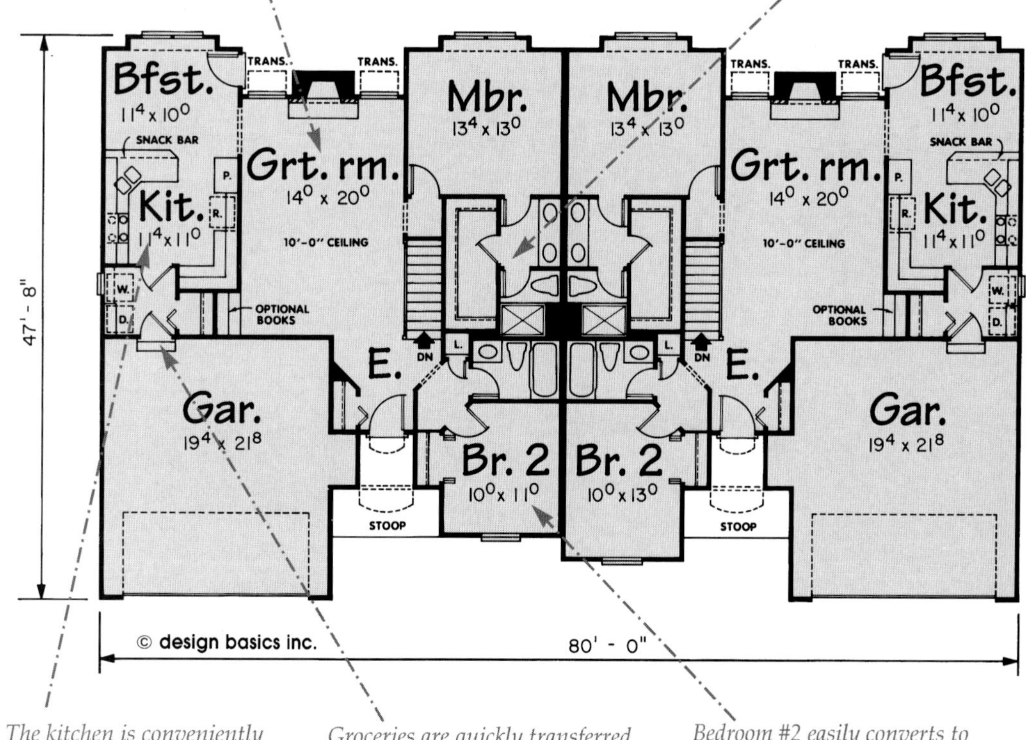

The kitchen is conveniently designed with immediate access to the laundry area.

Groceries are quickly transferred from car to kitchen.

Bedroom #2 easily converts to a den or home office.

Duplex Plan

Left Side: 1212 Sq. Ft.	Right Side: 1233 Sq. Ft.

#28A-8174 Plan Price $595

ADDITIONAL DUPLEX PLANS
are available from Design Basics. Call 1-800-947-7526 for information.

Situation

He has a bumper sticker on his car that says, "I'd rather be golfing." And if you know my husband, it speaks the truth. Seven days a week is not enough time on the golf course as far as he is concerned. If his company would let him he'd wear his golf shirts to work. He's hinted that his next investment will inevitably be a golf cart (and more than likely a new set of clubs). And our plans for a new home must have a place for it I'm told – and, of course, a view of a beautiful water hazard. . .

Solution

Perfect for a golf course lot, the Mansfield offers a three-car tandem drive-through garage (❷, at far right). It's the perfect place to keep a golf cart and have direct access to the course. The Comstock also offers a third stall that's conducive to storing a golf cart to drive straight out to the greens (❶, at right).

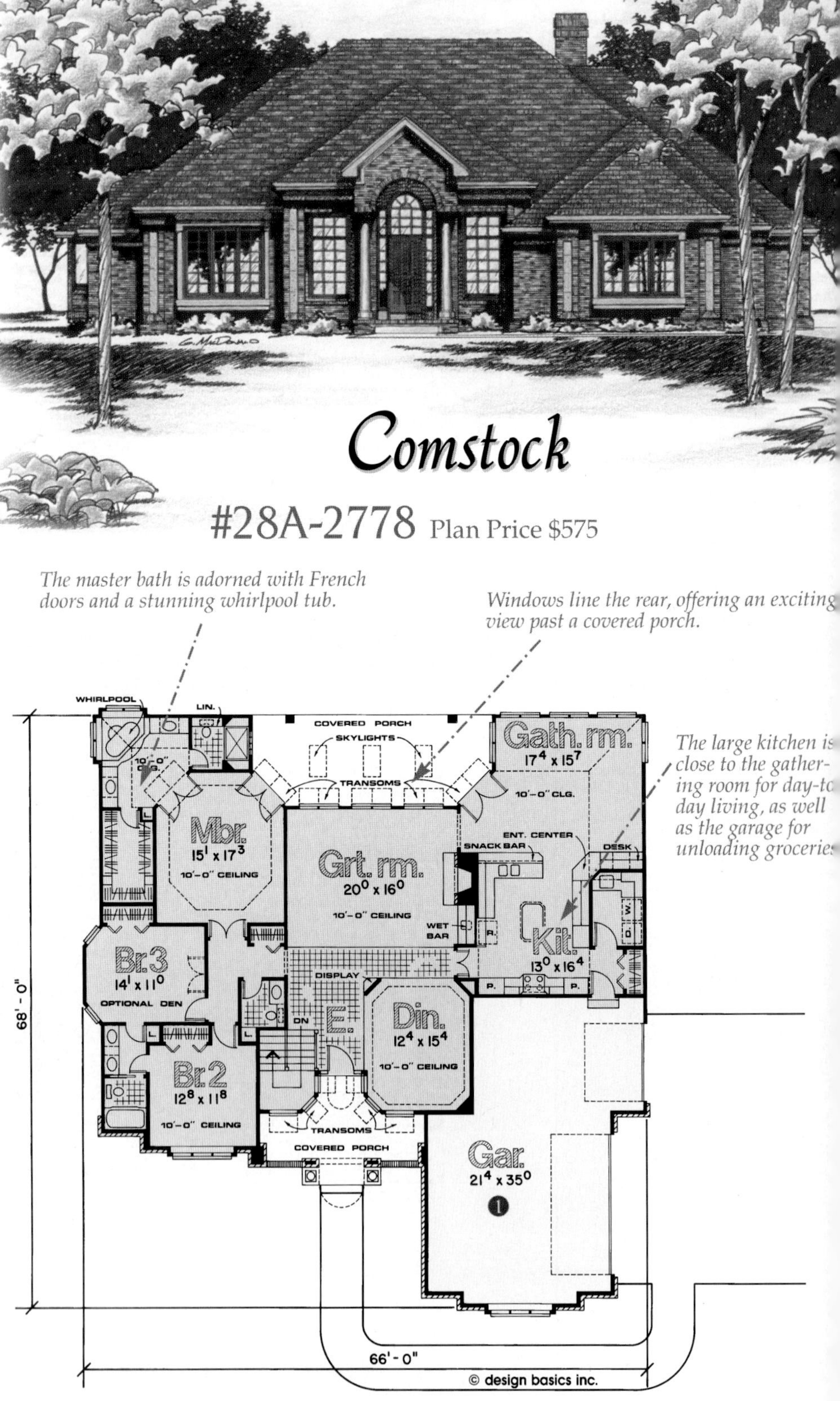

Comstock

#28A-2778 Plan Price $575

The master bath is adorned with French doors and a stunning whirlpool tub.

Windows line the rear, offering an exciting view past a covered porch.

The large kitchen is close to the gathering room for day-to-day living, as well as the garage for unloading groceries.

Total Square Feet: 2456 Sq. Ft.

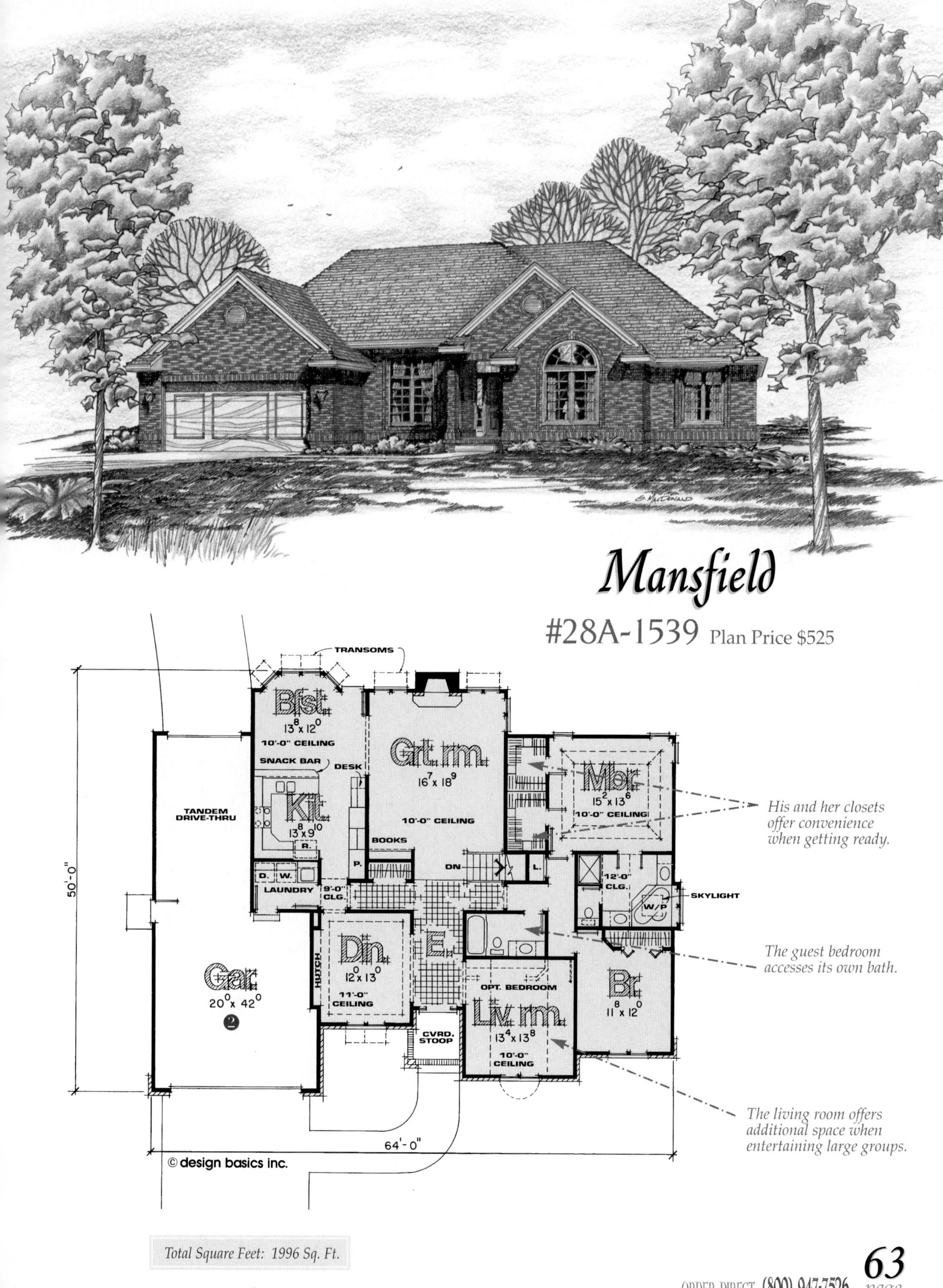

Mansfield

#28A-1539 Plan Price $525

His and her closets offer convenience when getting ready.

The guest bedroom accesses its own bath.

The living room offers additional space when entertaining large groups.

Total Square Feet: 1996 Sq. Ft.

OUTDOOR LIVING AREAS . . . *It seems nothing is more relaxing than kicking back with an iced drink out on a porch or patio. Outdoor living spaces have a way of helping us remove ourselves from our busy lives. The following plans reveal a variety of outdoor living spaces for those of us who consider them an essential part of our home. . .*

A TASTE OF GINGERBREAD

Main Floor: 1421 Sq. Ft.
Second Floor: 578 Sq. Ft.
Total Square Feet: 1999 Sq. Ft.

Andover

#28A-1863 Plan Price $525

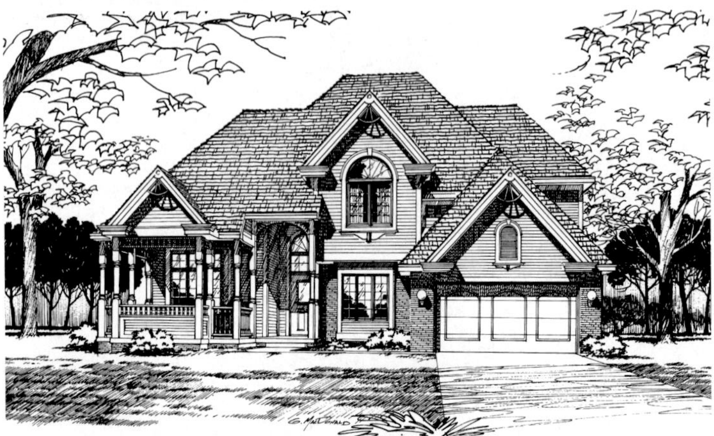

A see-thru fireplace brings a comfortable ambiance to meals in the breakfast area.

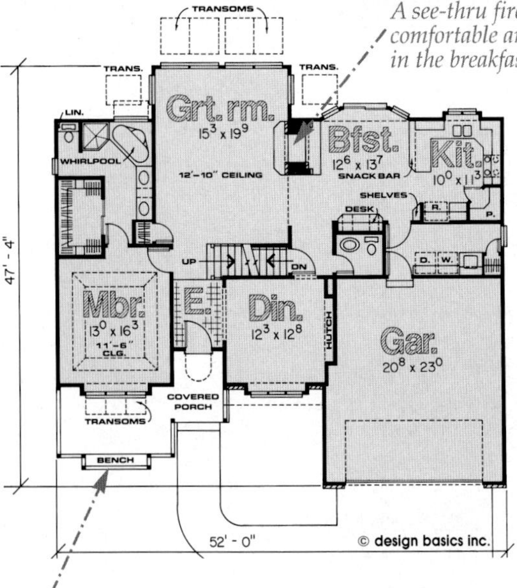

A built-in bench highlights the large front porch.

A large bonus room on the second floor can convert into a bedroom or office.

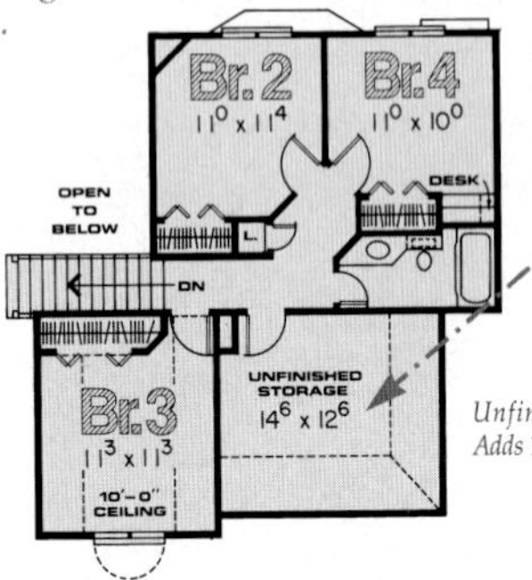

Unfinished Storage Adds 185 Square Feet

WIDE-OPEN SPACES

Main Floor: 2813 Sq. Ft.
Second Floor: 1091 Sq. Ft.
Total Square Feet: 3904 Sq. Ft.

Fairchild

#28A-2733 Plan Price $725

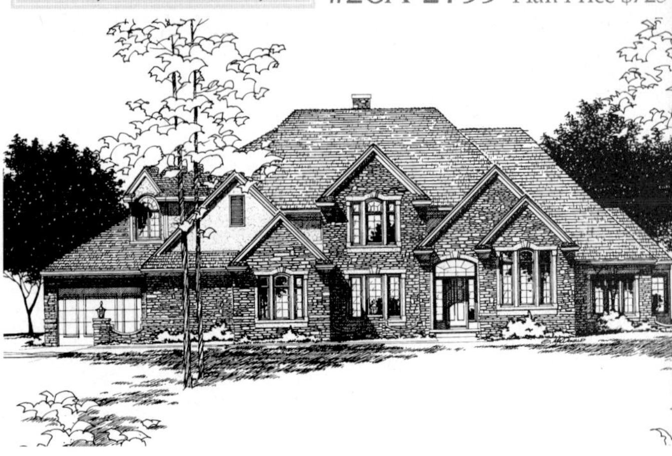

A long snack bar peninsula serves the informal breakfast area and family room.

A rear covered porch has access from the master bath and casual family area.

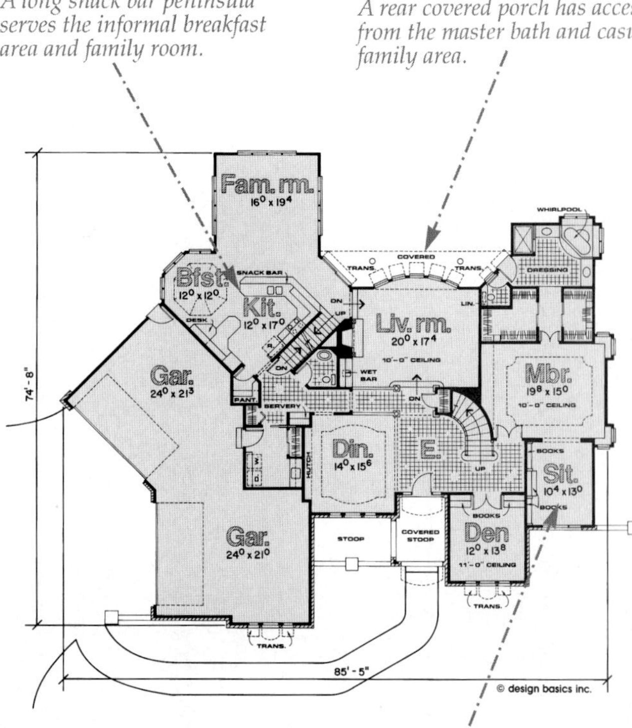

A sitting room accompanies the master suite and features built-in shelves for books or electronic equipment.

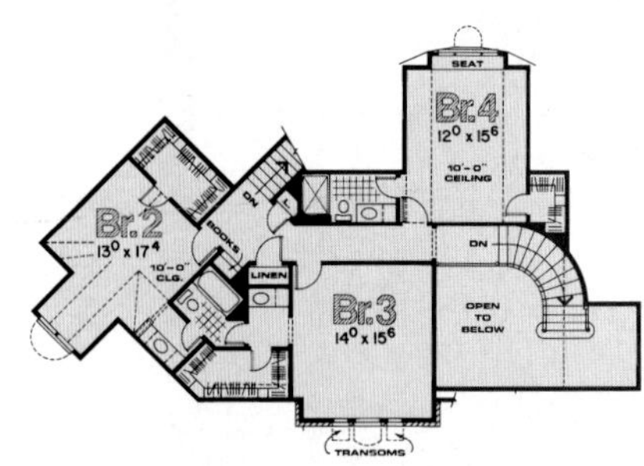

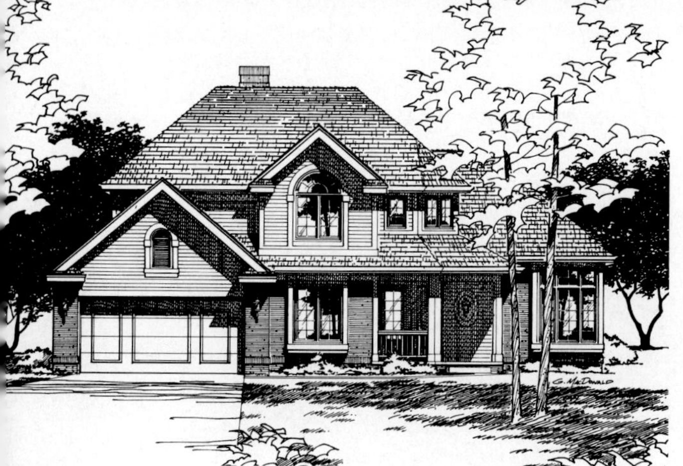

A PORCH WITH ALL THE RIGHT ANGLES

Main Floor: 1510 Sq. Ft.
Second Floor: 579 Sq. Ft.
Total Square Feet: 2089 Sq. Ft.

Sierra

#28A-2745 Plan Price $535

ows flood the great and breakfast area natural light.

A corner whirlpool tub and large walk-in closet complete the private master suite.

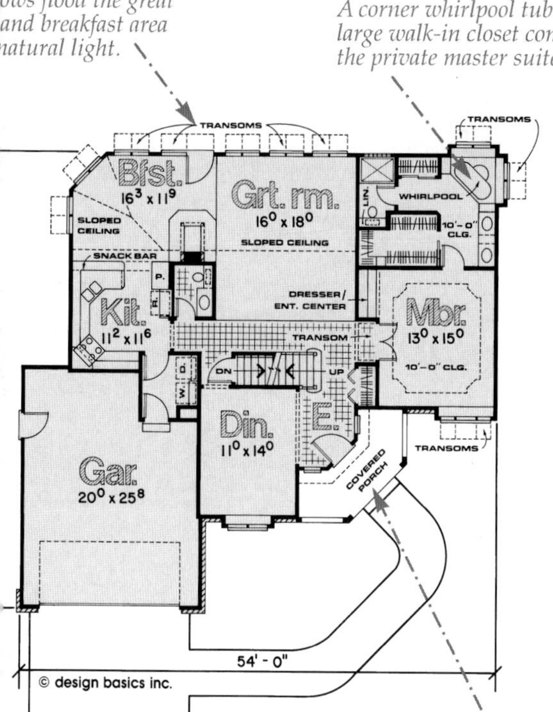

An angled porch welcomes a pair of chairs.

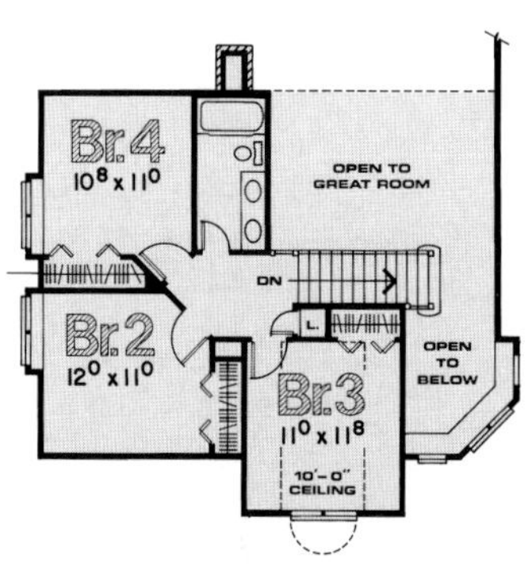

*A*CCESSIBLE BACK PORCHES

Main Floor: 2098 Sq. Ft.
Second Floor: 790 Sq. Ft.
Total Square Feet: 2888 Sq. Ft.

Gossard

#28A-3442 Plan Price $615

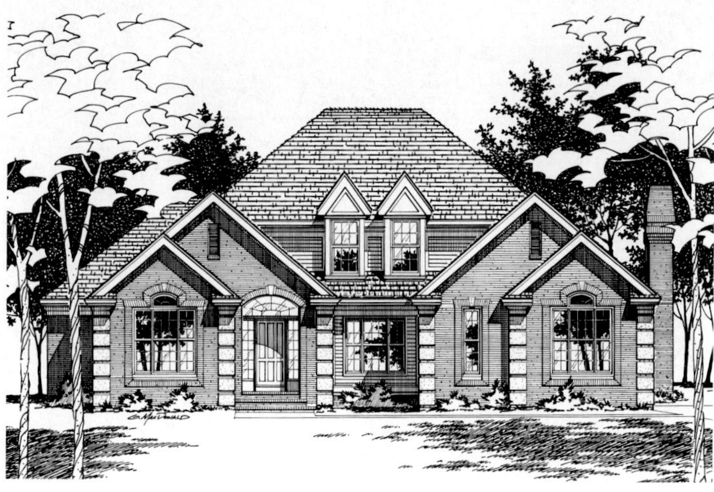

Two covered porches at the back of the home are accessible from the breakfast area and master suite.

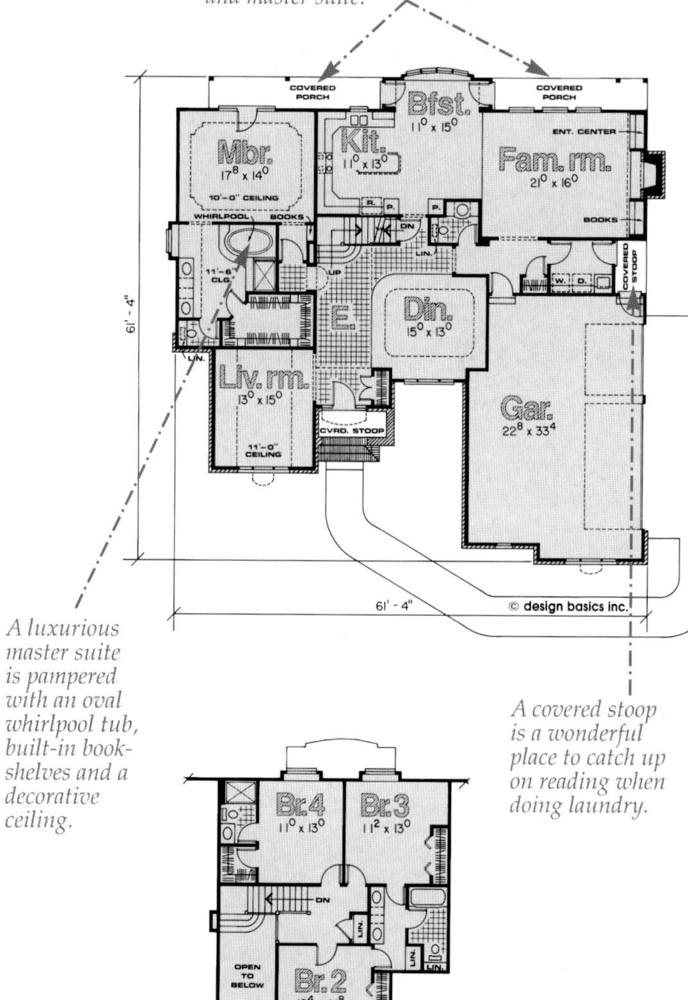

A luxurious master suite is pampered with an oval whirlpool tub, built-in bookshelves and a decorative ceiling.

A covered stoop is a wonderful place to catch up on reading when doing laundry.

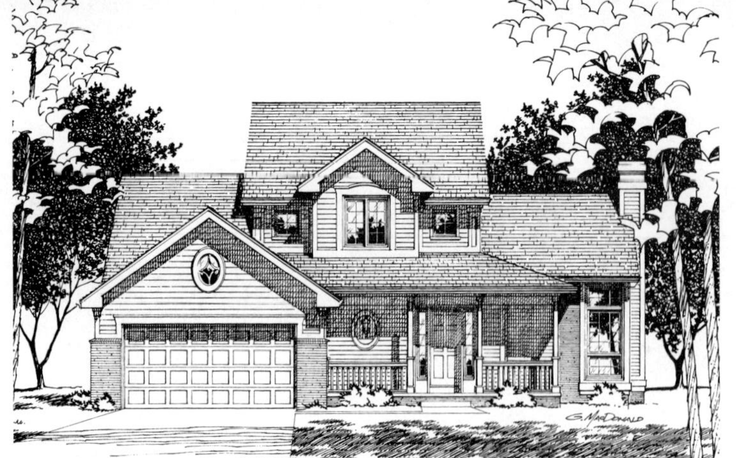

WRAPPED WITH CHARM

Main Floor: 1191 Sq. Ft.
Second Floor: 405 Sq. Ft.
Total Square Feet: 1596 Sq. Ft.

Bethany

#28A-3123 Plan Price $485

An angled hall secludes the master suite, featuring an illuminated whirlpool and large walk-in closet.

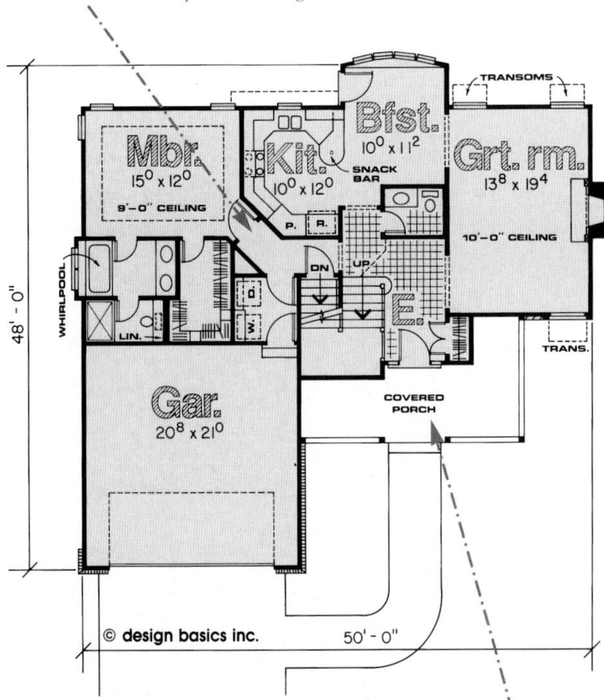

A second-floor balcony presents a charming view in the two-story entry.

The large front porch makes a wonderful alternative to the indoors on a pleasant day.

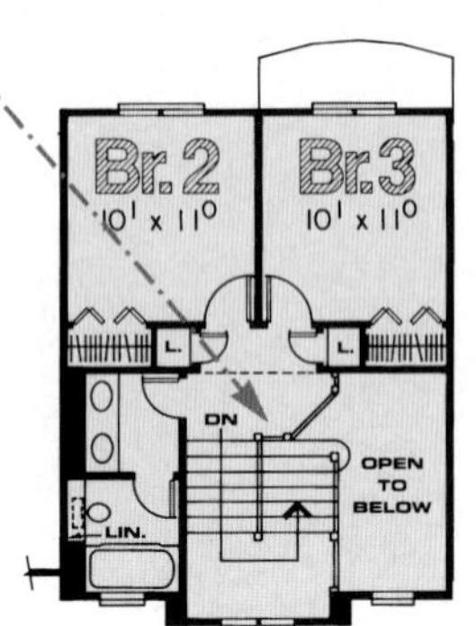

POTENTIAL LIVING SPACE

Main Floor: 1736 Sq. Ft.
Second Floor: 660 Sq. Ft.
Total Square Feet: 2396 Sq. Ft.

Bryant Woods

#28A-8041 Plan Price $465

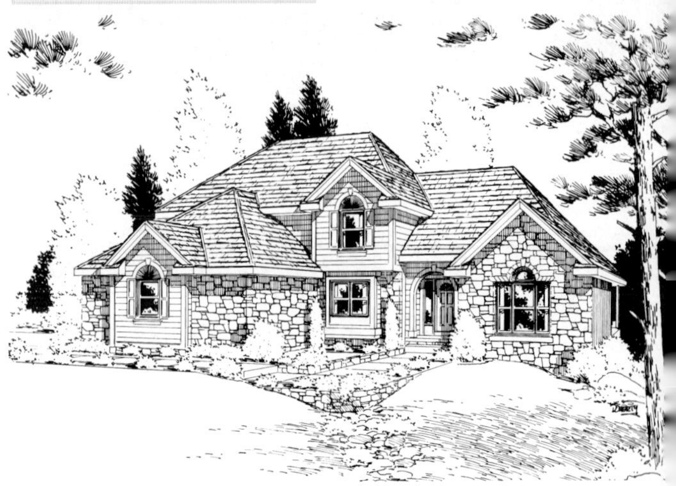

A see-thru fireplace warms both the great room and hearth room/kitchen.

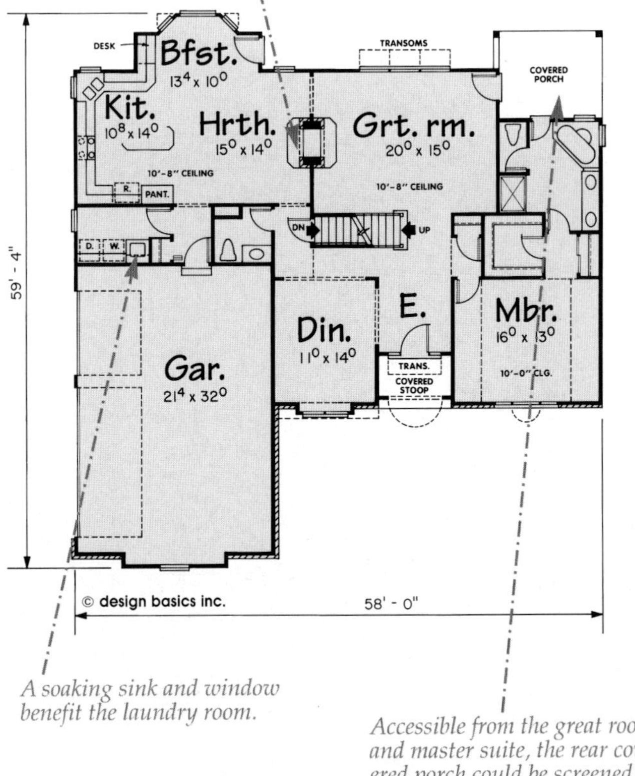

A soaking sink and window benefit the laundry room.

Accessible from the great room and master suite, the rear covered porch could be screened in for a three season room.

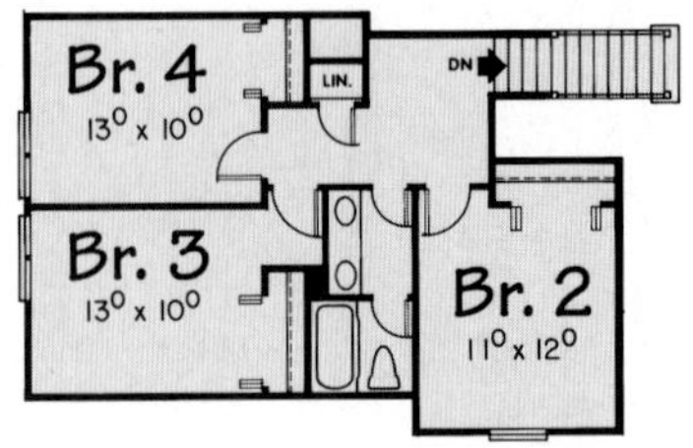

PRIVATE GET-AWAY

Main Floor: 1800 Sq. Ft.
Second Floor: 803 Sq. Ft.
Total Square Feet: 2603 Sq. Ft.

Rollins

#28A-2894 Plan Price $595

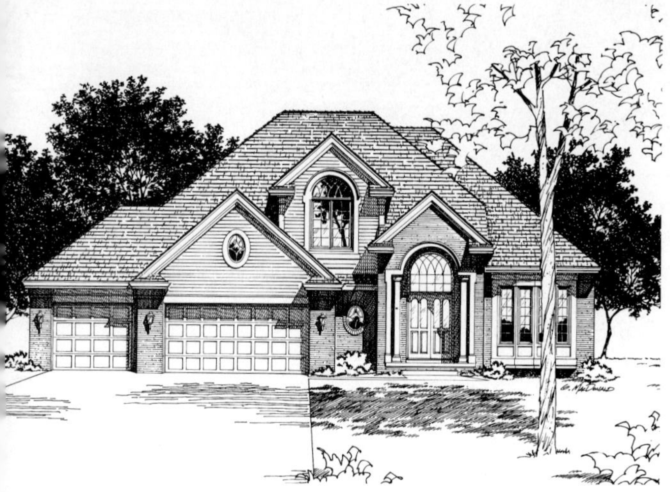

naster suite features access to a private ed porch - a great place to get away.

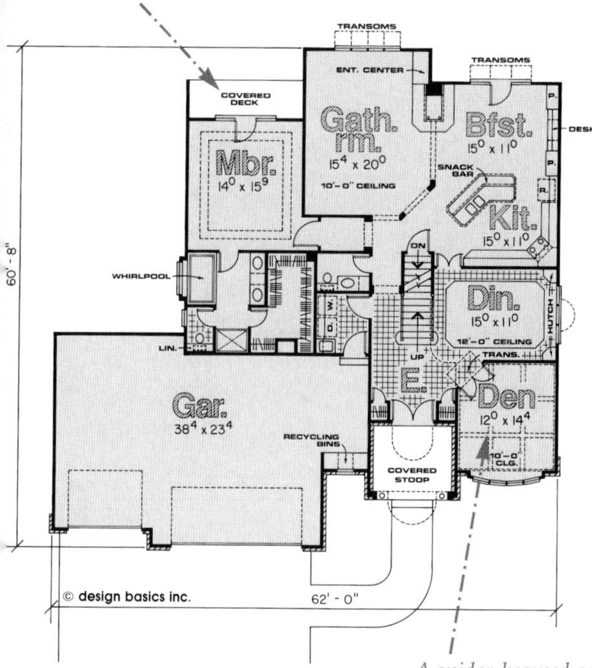

A spider-beamed ceiling and double doors highlight the den.

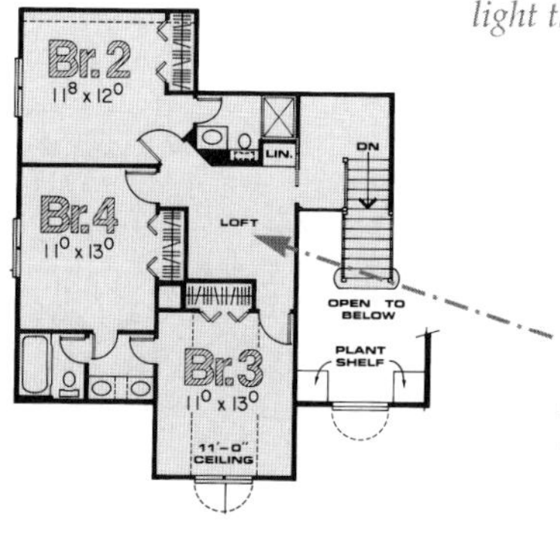

A second-floor loft is a great place for a homework area and the home computer.

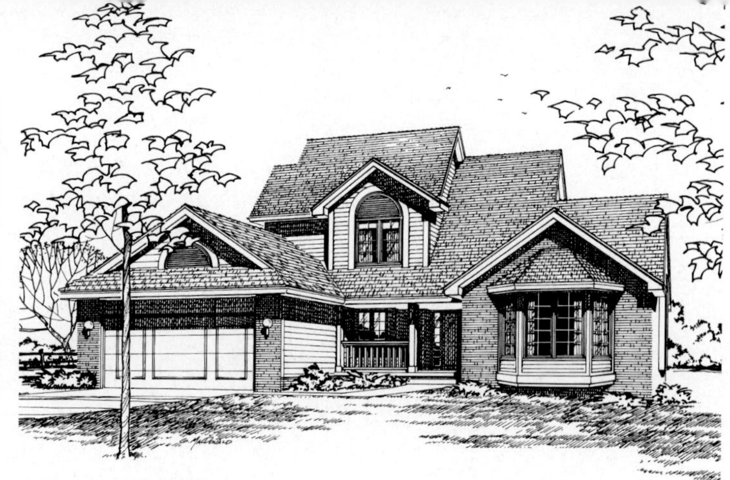

BACKYARD BARBECUE

Main Floor: 1306 Sq. Ft.
Second Floor: 425 Sq. Ft.
Total Square Feet: 1731 Sq. Ft.

Crescent

#28A-1734 Plan Price $505

A back patio is a great place to barbecue with easy access from the kitchen.

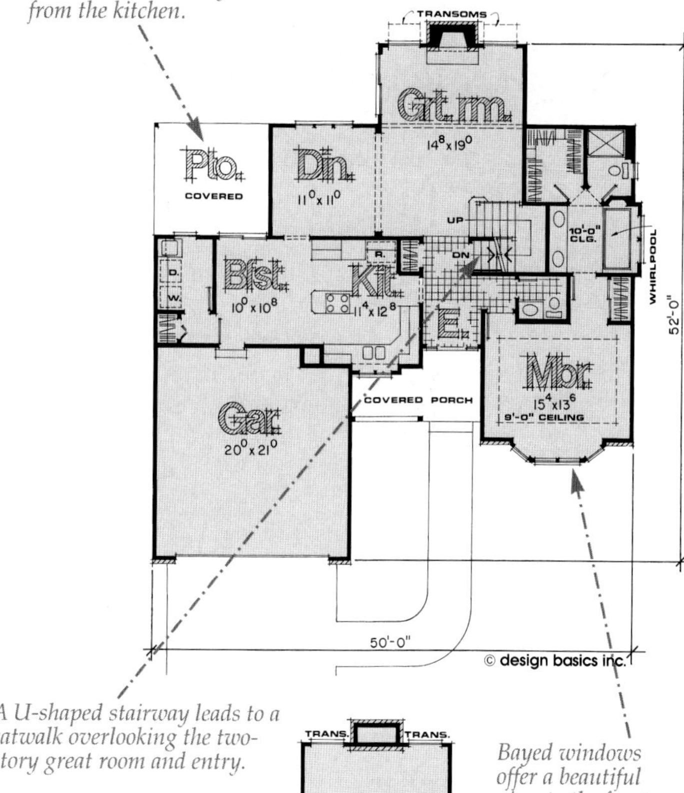

A U-shaped stairway leads to a catwalk overlooking the two-story great room and entry.

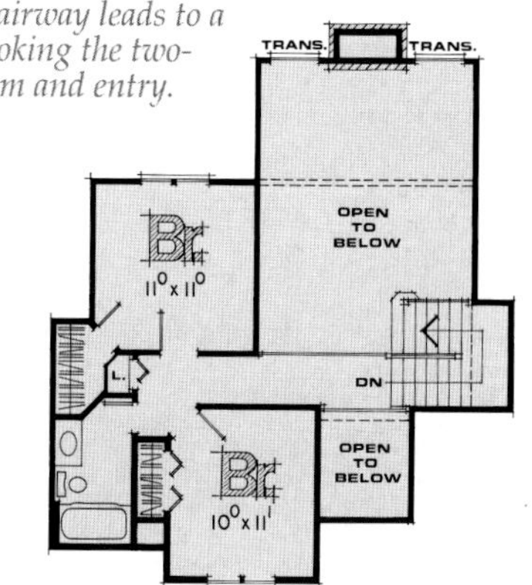

Bayed windows offer a beautiful view to the front in the master bedroom.

WELL-LIT SPACES . . . *Whether empty-nester, or not, everyone likes a place with an abundance of natural light. It makes any size room feel open and unrestricted. The following eight plans all provide unique places to enjoy the sunshine or take advantage of a beautiful view.*

WINDOWS FOR EVERY ROOM

Hillcrest

Main Floor: 1865 Sq. Ft.
Second Floor: 774 Sq. Ft.
Total Square Feet: 2639 Sq. Ft.

#28A-2649 Plan Price $595

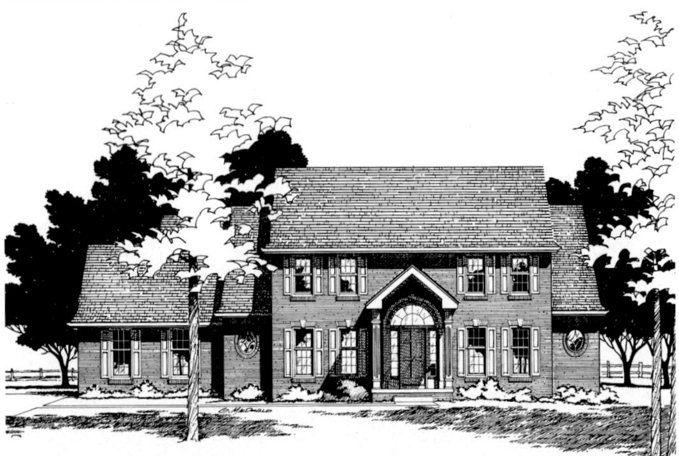

Tall double transom windows illuminate the comfortable breakfast area.

The master bath is brightened by a large transom window over the whirlpool tub.

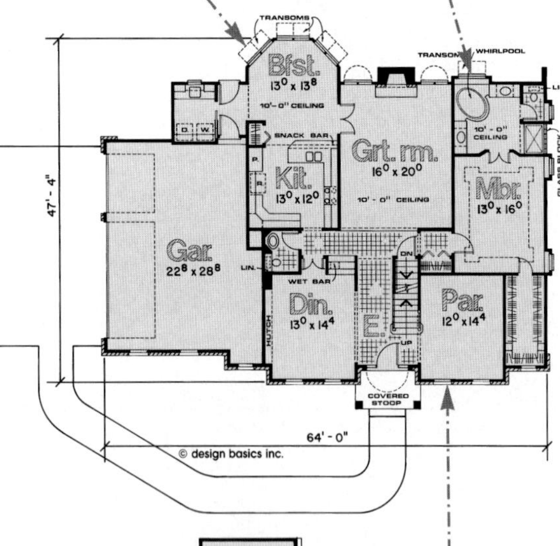

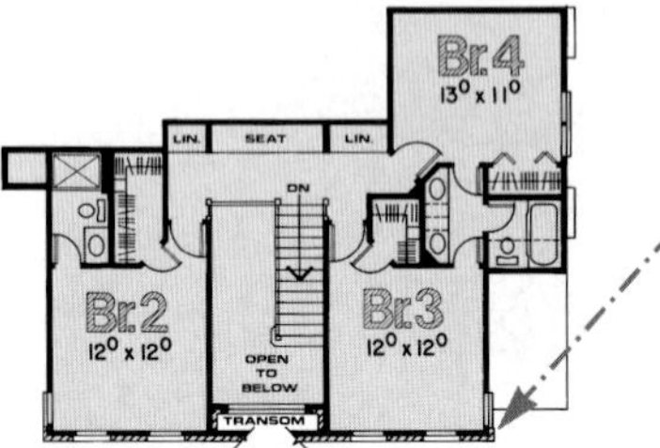

Twin double-hung windows bring sophistication and light to the formal rooms and two secondary bedrooms.

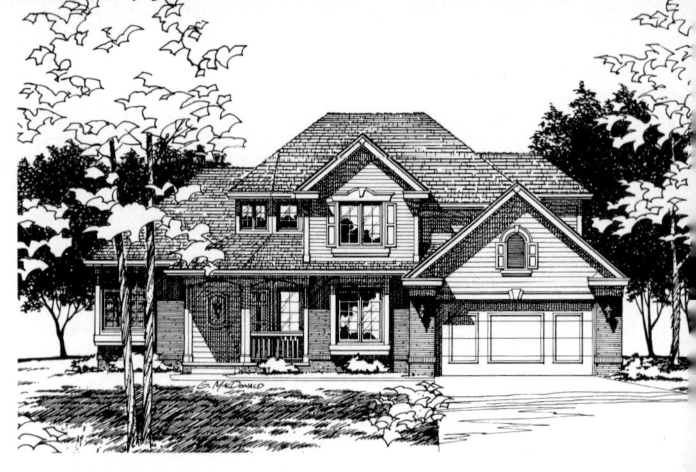

BRIGHT MASTER BATH

Eldorado

Main Floor: 1413 Sq. Ft.
Second Floor: 563 Sq. Ft.
Total Square Feet: 1976 Sq. Ft.

#28A-2719 Plan Price $525

Tall windows with transoms offer striking views from the great room and kitchen/dinette.

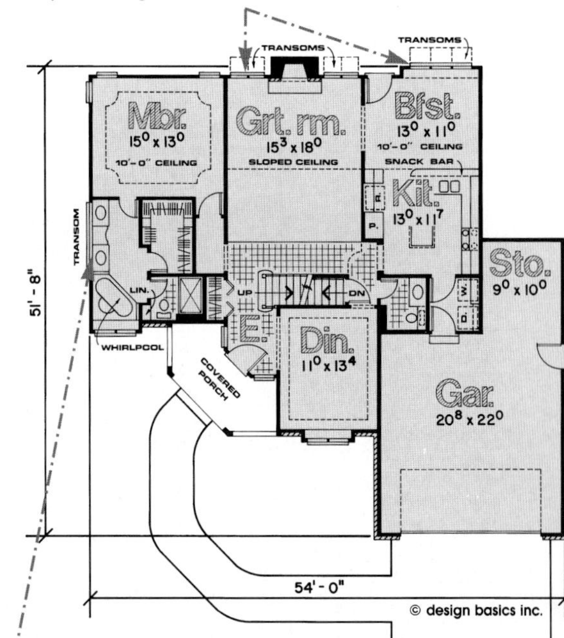

A double window and transom bring a sense of openness to the master bath.

A set of bayed windows with display ledge decorates the two-story entry.

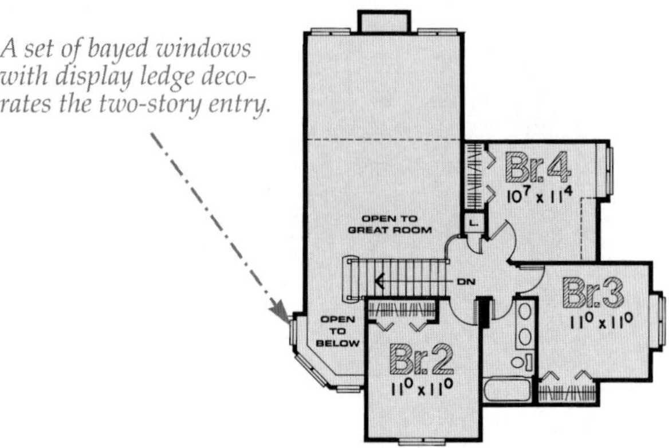

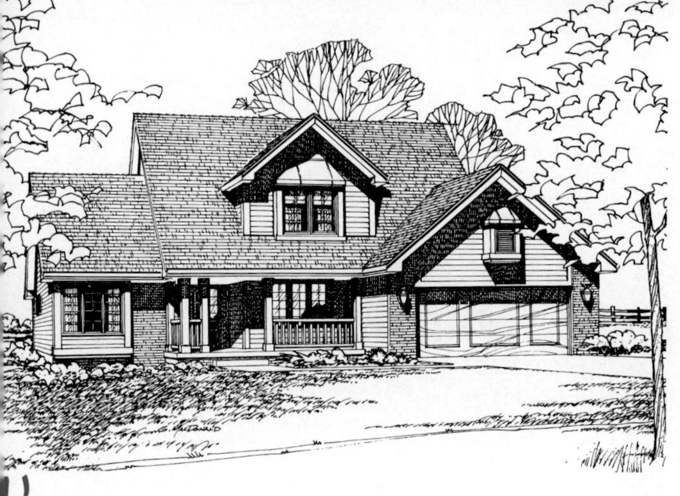

IEWS TO THE REAR

Main Floor: 1421 Sq. Ft.
Second Floor: 448 Sq. Ft.
Total Square Feet: 1869 Sq. Ft.

Trenton

#28A-1330 Plan Price $515

A see-thru fireplace provides warmth in the bright kitchen/breakfast area.

vindows wrapping the great offer the opportunity to enjoy utiful view to the back.

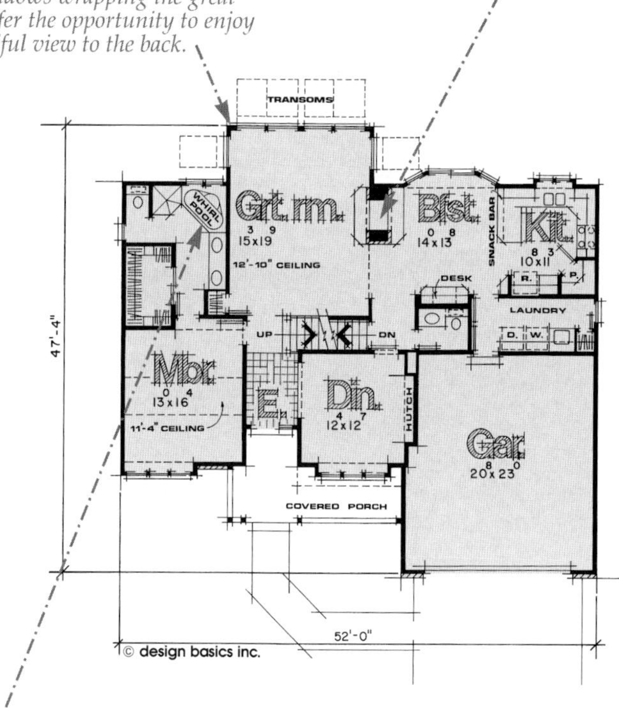

master suite is complemented ı a sunny whirlpool tub and -angled shower.

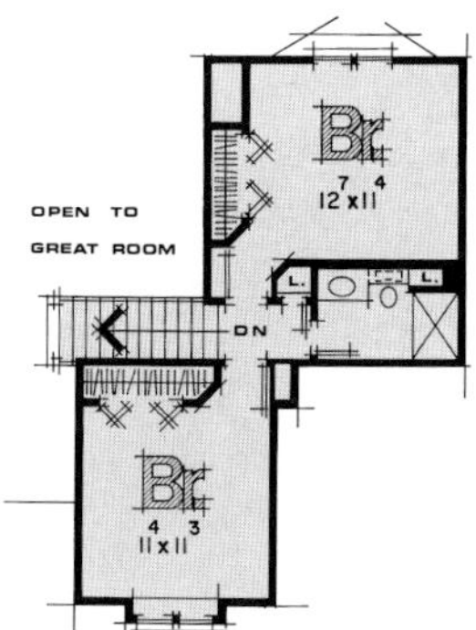

SUNNY MASTER SUITE

Main Floor: 1972 Sq. Ft.
Second Floor: 893 Sq. Ft.
Total Square Feet: 2865 Sq. Ft.

Remington

#28A-1486 Plan Price $615

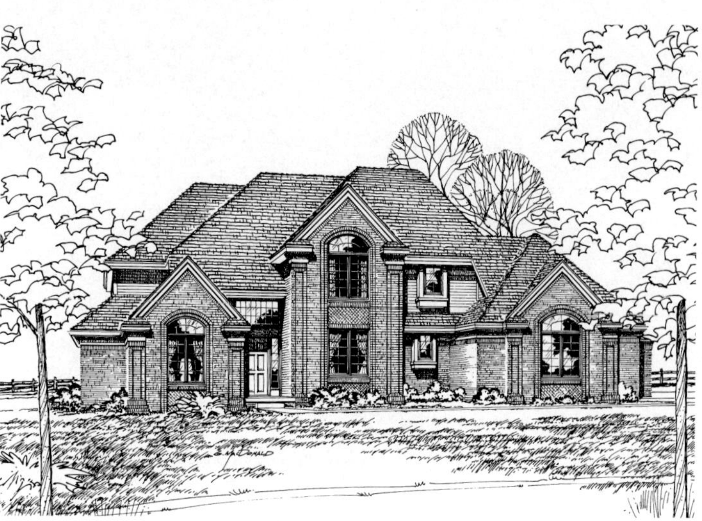

Bowed windows help brighten the master suite, enhanced with a tiered ceiling.

A valley cathedral accentuates four tall windows in the great room.

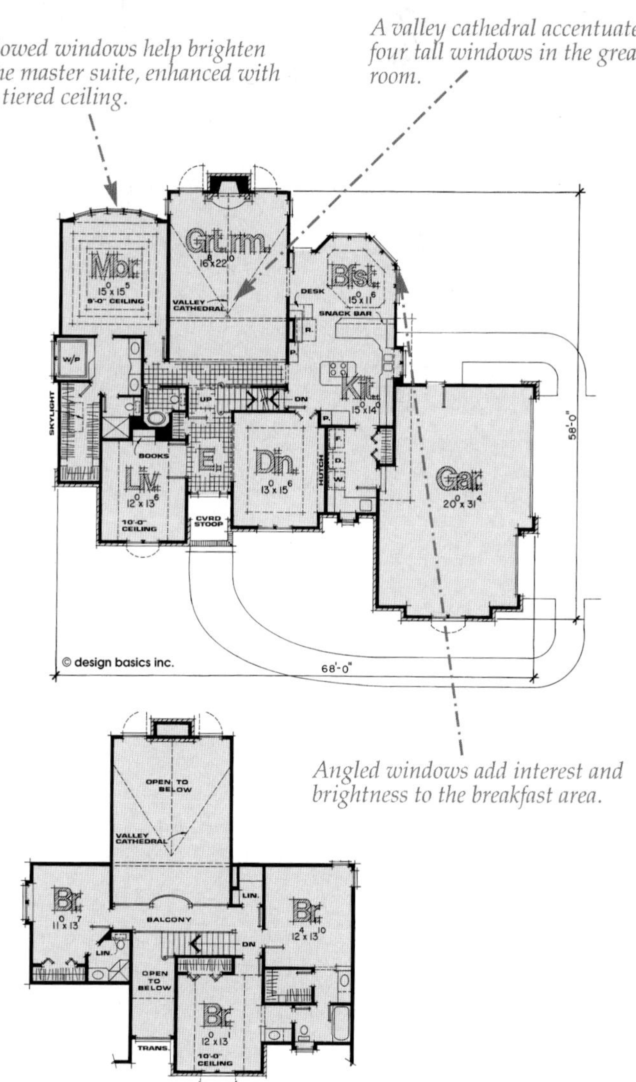

Angled windows add interest and brightness to the breakfast area.

Flooded with Light

Bermier

Main Floor: 1297 Sq. Ft.
Second Floor: 558 Sq. Ft.
Total Square Feet: 1855 Sq. Ft.

#28A-2236 Plan Price $515

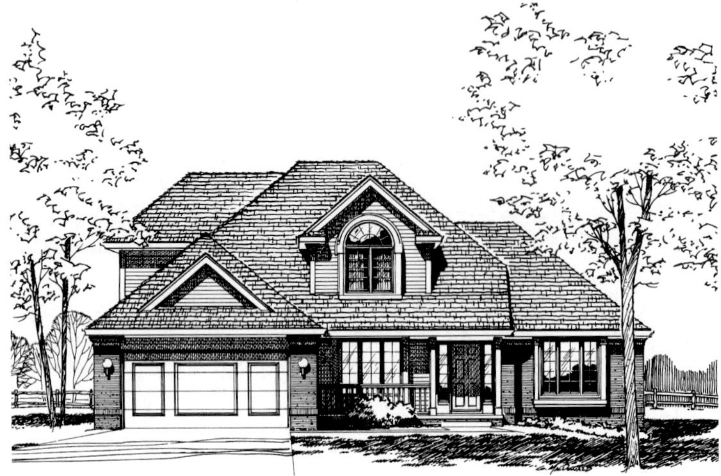

Four tall windows wrap the great room in natural light.

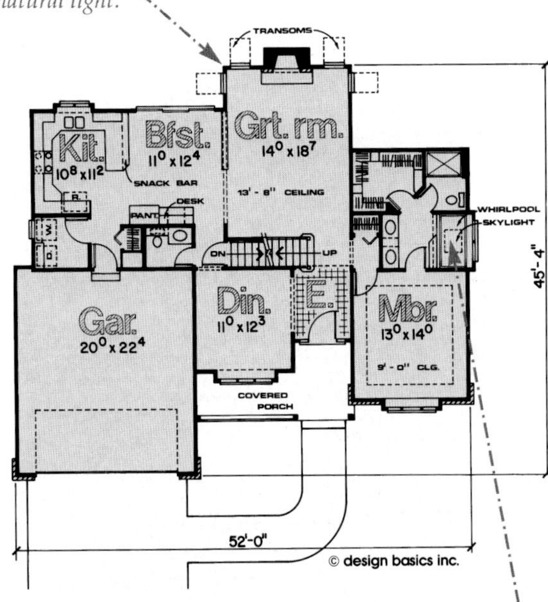

A skylight floods the master bath with sunshine.

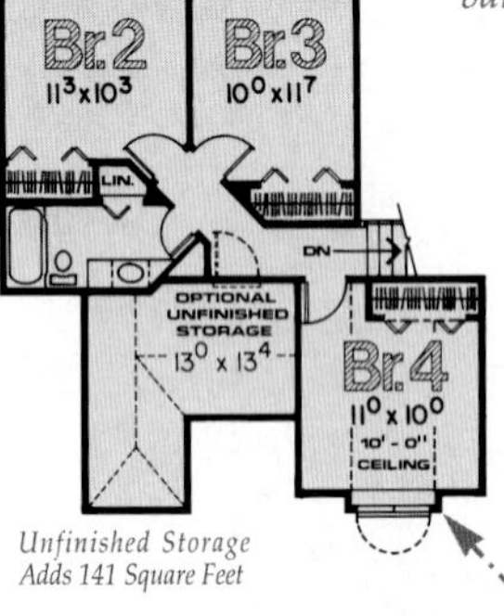

Unfinished Storage Adds 141 Square Feet

An arched window and volume ceiling add spaciousness to bedroom #4.

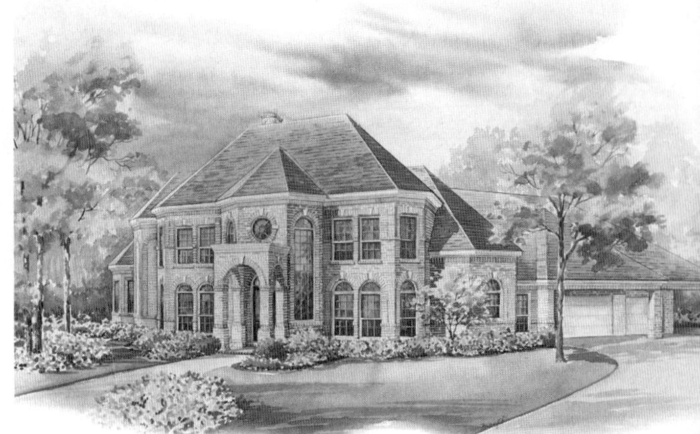

Ascend in Sunshine

Oak Grove Estat

#28A-9143 Plan Price $7

Main Floor: 2274 Sq. Ft.
Second Floor: 1476 Sq. Ft.
Total Square Feet: 3750 Sq. Ft.

Both the master suite and great room enjoy luminous views to the back.

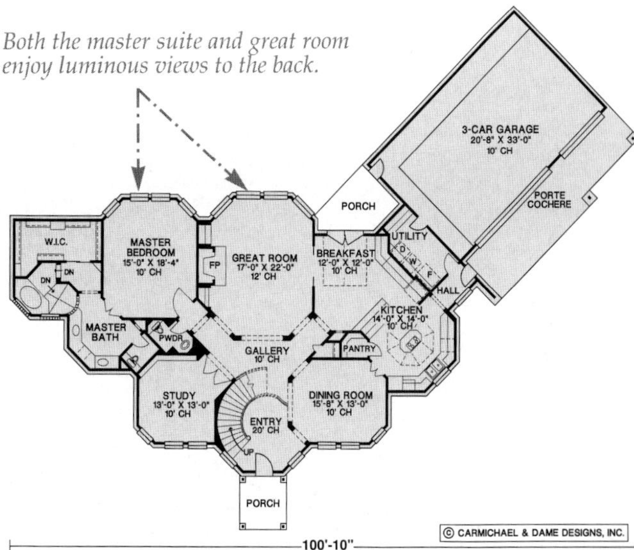

If using basement - dimensions changed to 105' 7" x 84' 9"

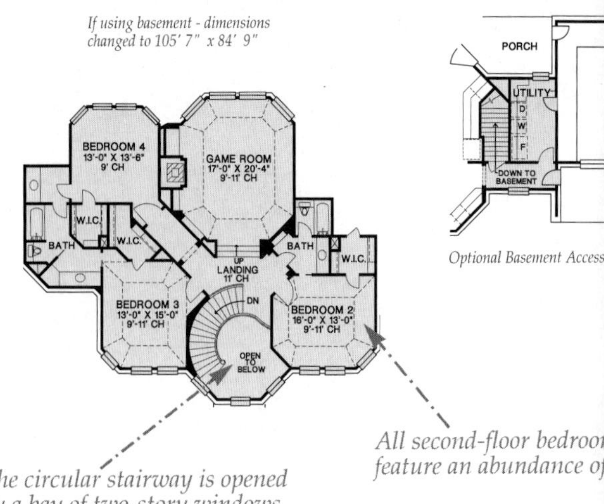

Optional Basement Access

The circular stairway is opened by a bay of two-story windows.

All second-floor bedroo feature an abundance o

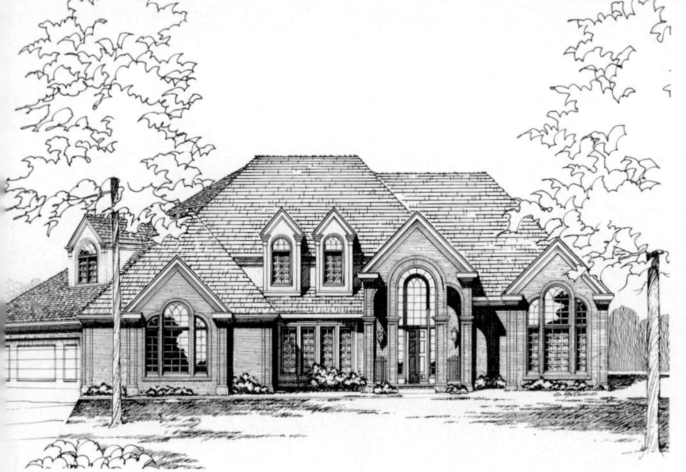

ELEGANT, AIRY ENTRY

Main Floor: 2617 Sq. Ft.
Second Floor: 1072 Sq. Ft.
Total Square Feet: 3689 Sq. Ft.

Le Grand

#28A-2218 Plan Price $695

Helping to brighten the master bath, patio doors lead to a covered porch.

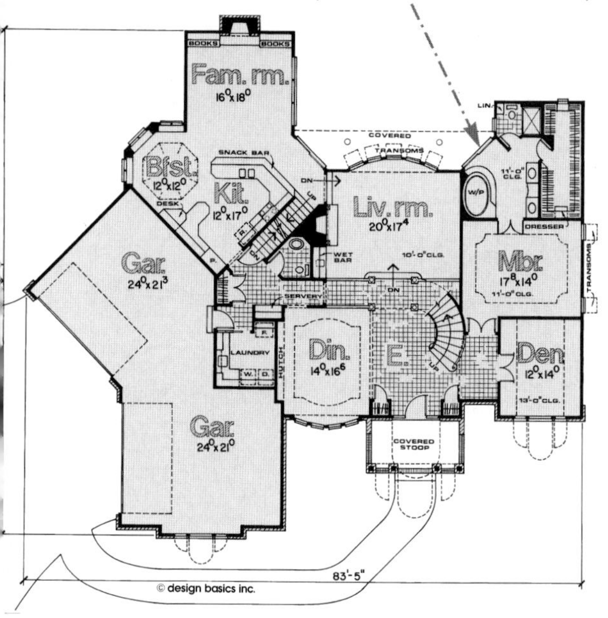

The two-story entry is immediately illuminated by a double-arched transom above the door.

…ped ceiling and …d window create …st in bedroom #2.

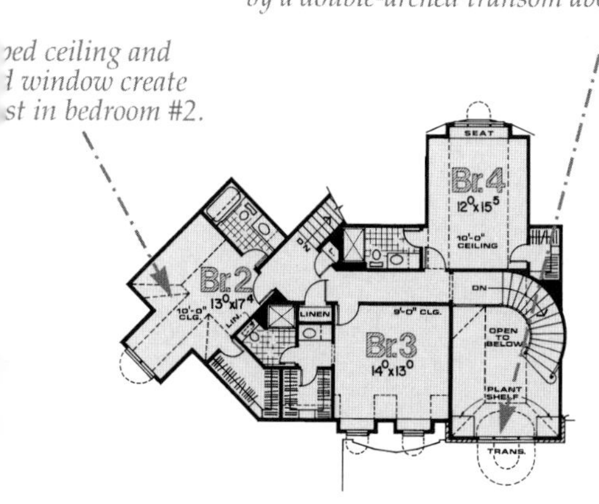

A GREAT ROOM WITH GREAT VIEWS

Main Floor: 1327 Sq. Ft.
Second Floor: 518 Sq. Ft.
Total Square Feet: 1845 Sq. Ft.

Ohern

#28A-2569 Plan Price $515

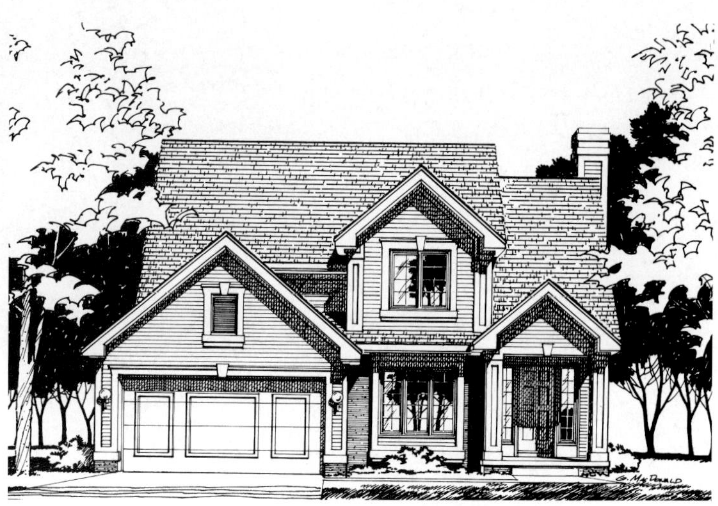

Natural light floods the volume great room through stunning windows with transoms.

A boxed, triple-wide window frames a lovely view to the rear in the master bedroom.

Three secondary bedrooms are secluded from main-floor activity.

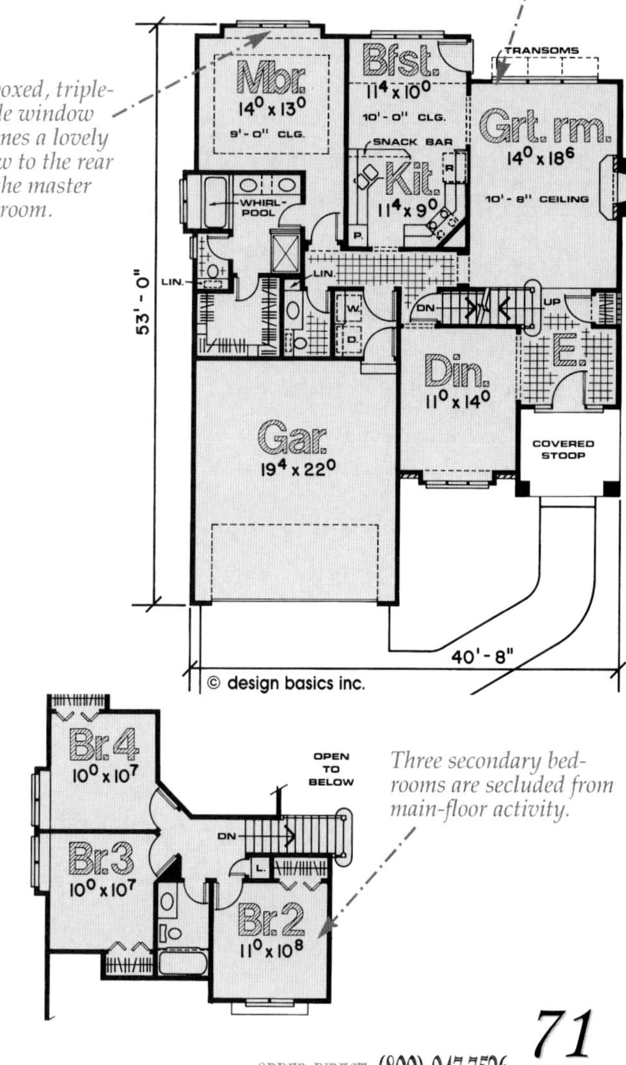

There were two types of people I knew about as a nine-year-old. There were city kids, and there were farm kids. And more than anything in the world, I wanted to be a city kid.

Growing up on our farm in central Kansas was achingly repressive to me. Staring out my bedroom window watching a pickup truck leave a cloud of dust along the country road near our home, I would often think to myself, "Wouldn't it be wonderful to live in town? If we lived in town we wouldn't have to can vegetables, gather eggs, milk cows or sew our own clothes. We could wear city clothes and play with our friends right across the street." It was the "perfection" of everything in towns that fascinated my nine-year-old mind. Neat rows of houses. The nearby five-and-dime. It all made sense to me. Churn your own butter? Why bother? I wanted cool, clean sidewalks to show me around and the heels of my store-bought shoes to click all the way to school.

If we lived in town we wouldn't have to can vegetables, gather eggs, milk cows or sew our own clothes.

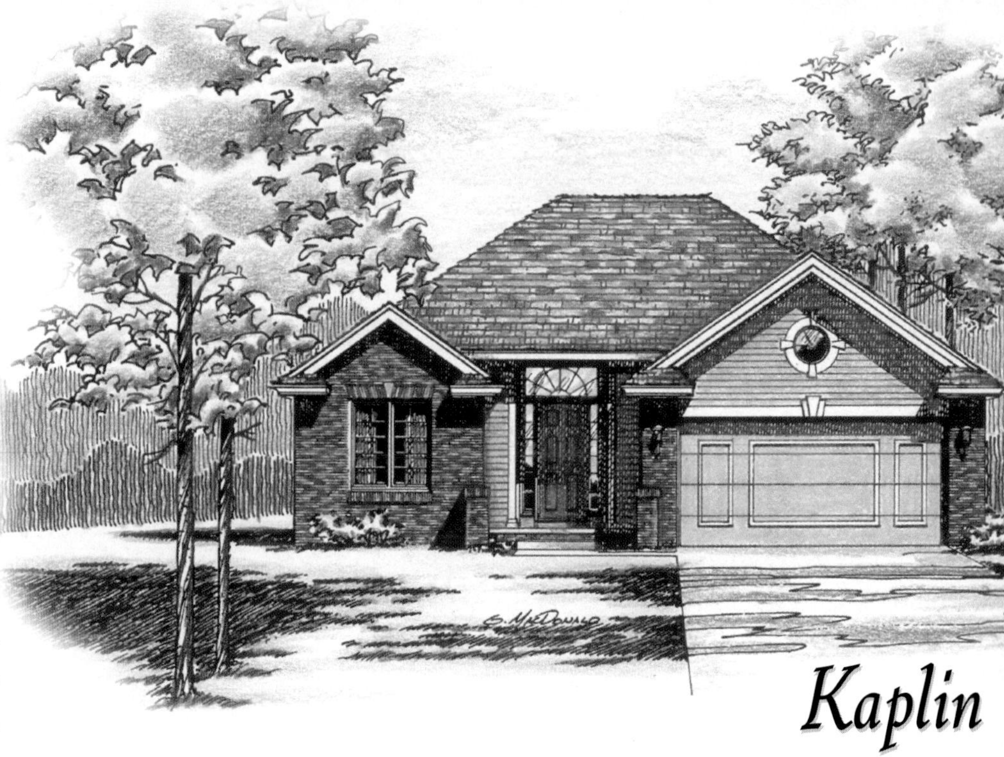

Kaplin

#28A-1963 Plan Price $465

Total Square Feet: 1347 Sq. Ft.

The secluded master suite has a large window to take advantage of an inviting view to the back.

The close proximity of the living areas fosters livability and efficiency in daily traffic flow.

Bedroom #3 easily converts into a den or hobby room.

Mbr. 13³ x 13⁰ 9'-4" CLG.
Skylight
W/P
B.
Transoms
Grt. rm. 14⁰ x 20⁰ 10'-0" Ceiling
Bfst. 12⁰ x 10⁰
Snack Bar
Kit. 12⁰ x 11²
R.
W.
D.
P.
Opt. Den
Br. 3 10⁰ x 10⁰
DN
E.
L.
Cvrd. Stoop
Br. 2 10⁰ x 10⁰
Gar. 19⁴ x 22⁴
54'-0"
42'-0"

© design basics inc.

Extra space in the garage leaves plenty of room for a garden center or work bench.

design basics inc. HOME PLAN DESIGN SERVICE

Instead, I had to settle for a dreadfully long gravel lane that my brothers and sisters and I would run down to catch the bus for a dreadfully long ride to school.

So, as soon as I graduated from Burns High School, I packed my bags and headed for college in the big city.

Those nine-year-old dreams came true. I got married and had children, making a life in suburbia with my loving husband. I now live near the grocery store and gas station in a neighborhood of similar-looking houses. I've lived the city life. But I'm 51 years old now. My children are gone. And I have come to the realization that ever since I left home for bigger and better things, I've been slowly returning to it. The more I thought I wanted a change, the more I found myself drawn back to the farm - a place that gave me the real meaning of home.

Oh, how my nine-year-old self would loath me now, thinking I've sold out. But that younger self hadn't tried to forget the taste of the raw beans we snapped on summer nights. How could she have possibly understood the way in which a sky full of stars and the cool of a front porch would stick with a person? I often find myself gazing upward on my front stoop in a needy remembrance.

My nine-year-old self would scoff at the vegetable garden I've had my whole married life. "What

cont'd on next page

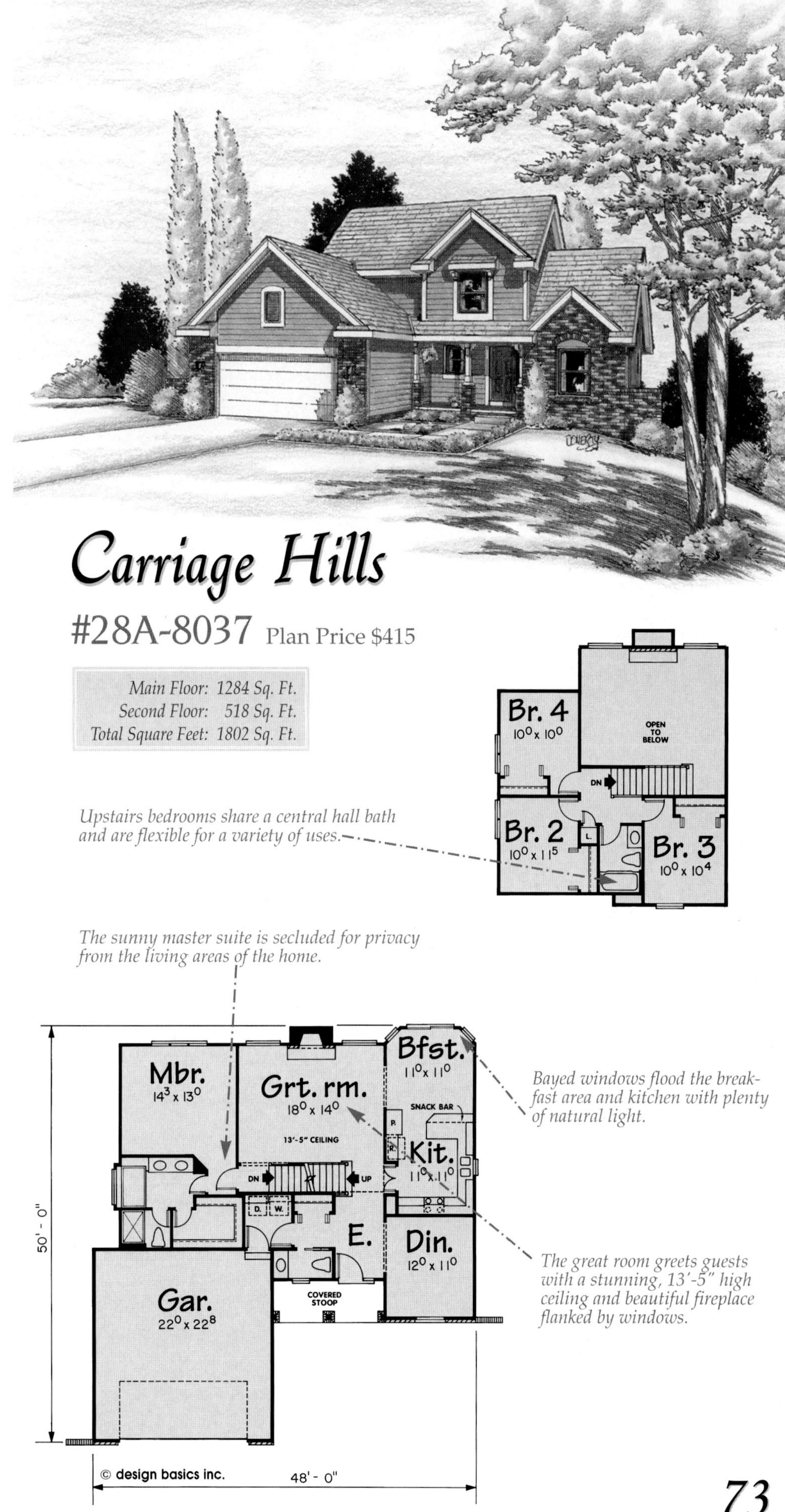

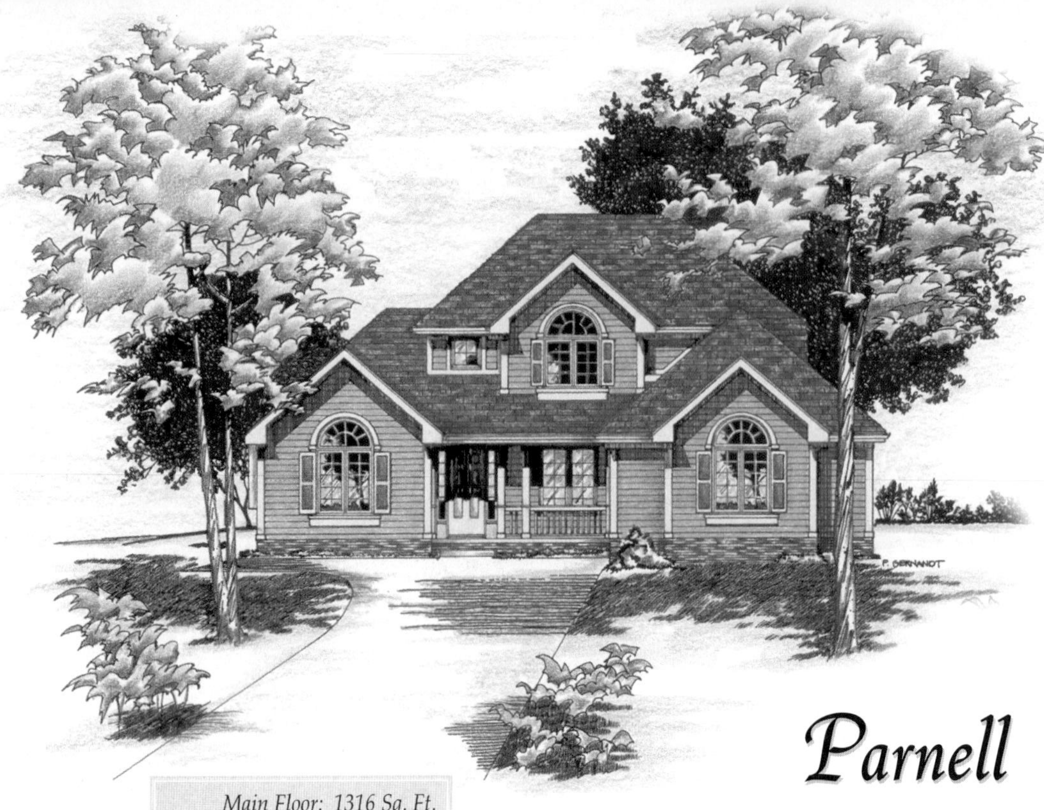

Parnell

Main Floor: 1316 Sq. Ft.
Second Floor: 396 Sq. Ft.
Total Square Feet: 1712 Sq. Ft.

#28A-3089 Plan Price $505

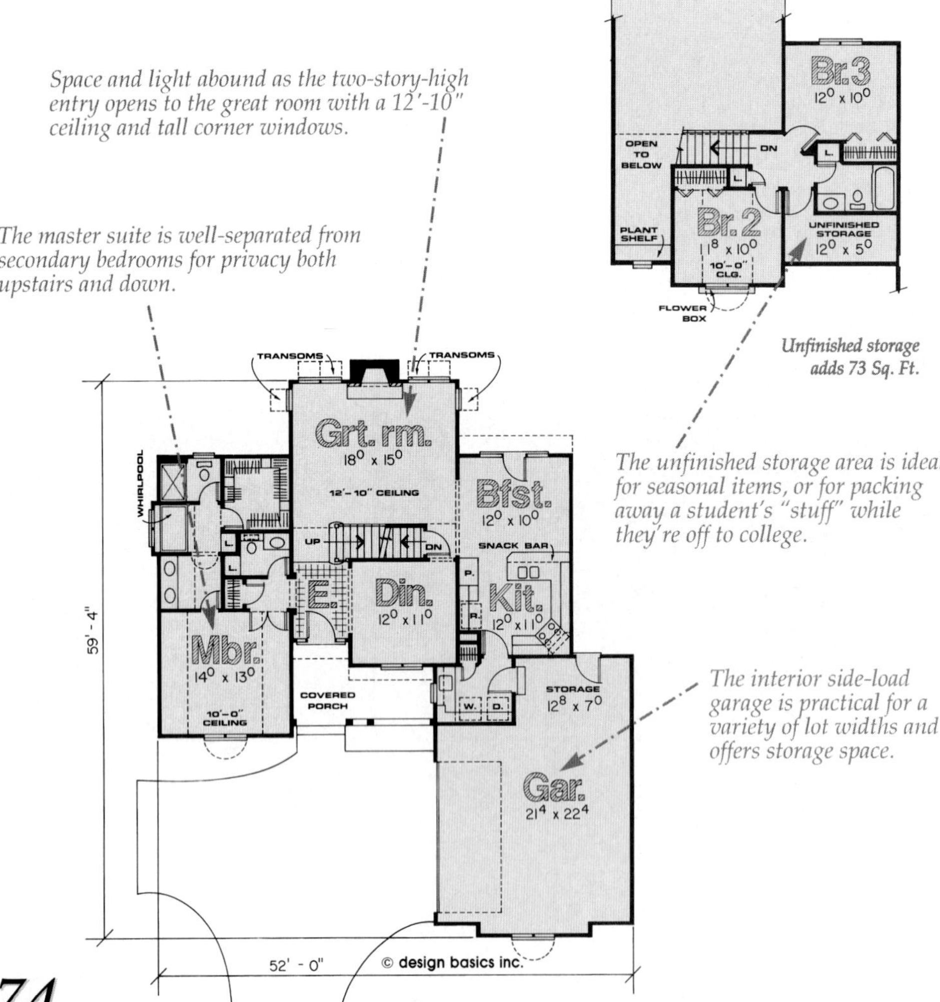

Space and light abound as the two-story-high entry opens to the great room with a 12'-10" ceiling and tall corner windows.

The master suite is well-separated from secondary bedrooms for privacy both upstairs and down.

Unfinished storage adds 73 Sq. Ft.

The unfinished storage area is ideal for seasonal items, or for packing away a student's "stuff" while they're off to college.

The interior side-load garage is practical for a variety of lot widths and offers storage space.

How could she have possibly understood the way in which a sky full of stars and the cool of a front porch would stick with a person.

are you doing?" she would say. "What about the convenience of the grocery store, with the pretty rows of neatly stacked fruits and vegetables? No work. No hassle. Remember?"

My nine-year-old mind could not have possibly believed the longing I would feel for my mother's cedar closet where we stored the winter clothes and her sewing room where she taught me the elegant art of needle and thread. It was a longing that eventually resulted in building the cedar closet we have in our basement and the conversion of our children's playroom into my sewing room. She could not have understood how I delve into making clothes and blankets for my new grandchild. Sewing a refuge? Therapy? What about the neatly placed store-bought dresses my nine-year old self could only admire? "With layers and layers of delicate ruffles," I hear her remind me. "What about the beautiful, perfect ruffles!"

Yet, deep down I think that if she'd truly known she'd have to one day give it all up, she'd take the farm with her to the city and settle for something in between, as I have.

cont'd on next page

design basics inc. HOME PLAN DESIGN SERVICE

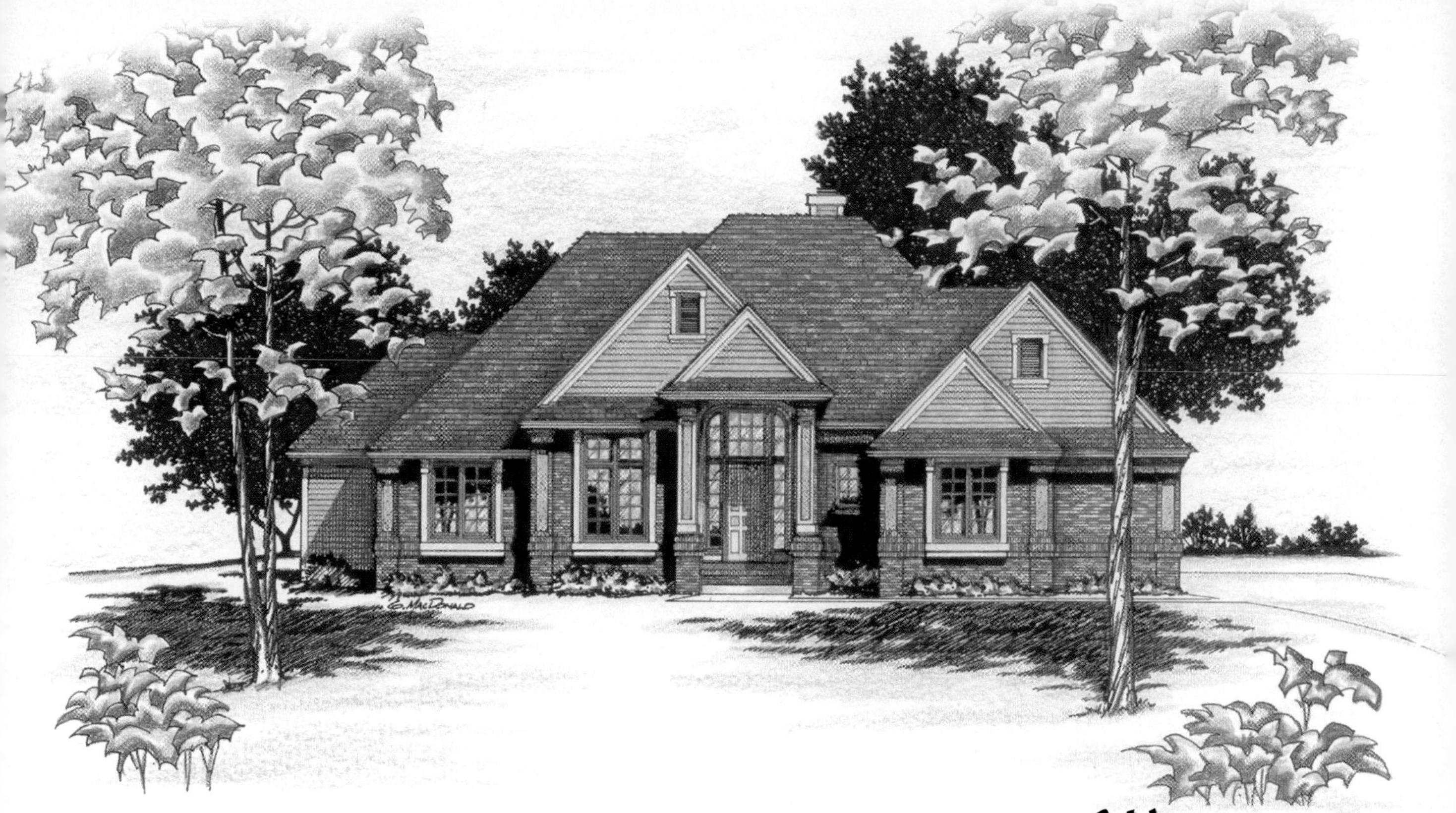

Wrenwood

#28A-3005 Plan Price $545

Total Square Feet: 2186 Sq. Ft.

A luxurious master suite features a two-person shower with built-in seats.

The kitchen is great for casual entertaining with a wet bar, large island cooktop, snack bar, and convenient access to the eating areas.

A room just off the kitchen is perfect for the home computer, a walk-in pantry, or extra storage.

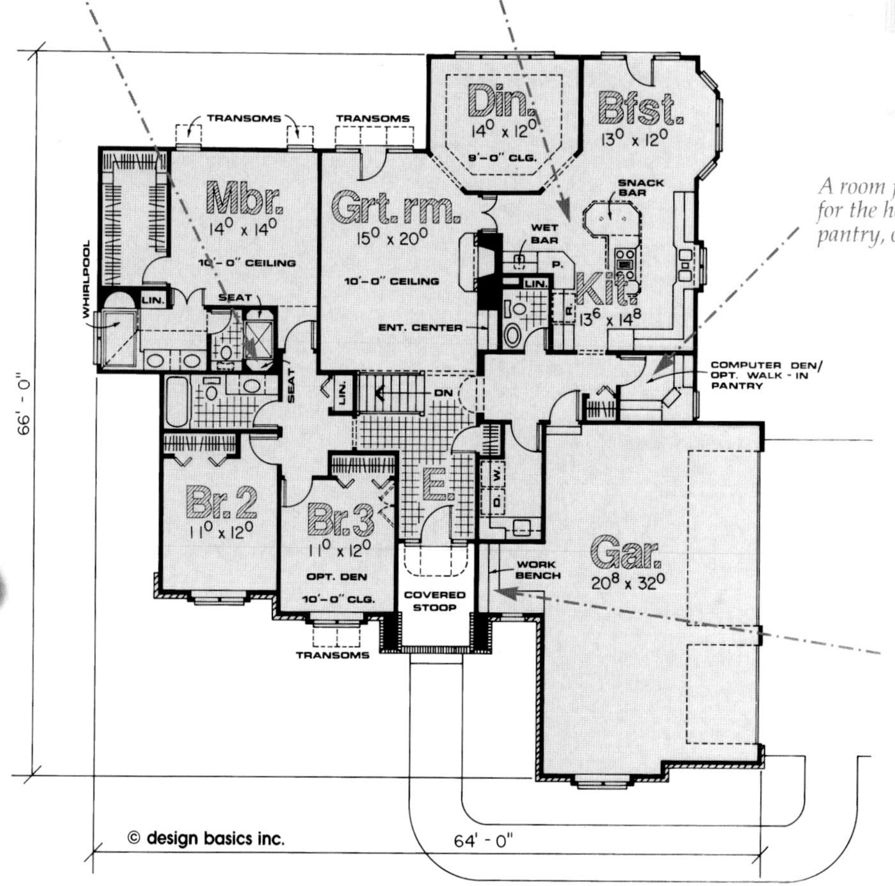

A well-lit work bench in the garage makes it easy to work on projects for home or hobby.

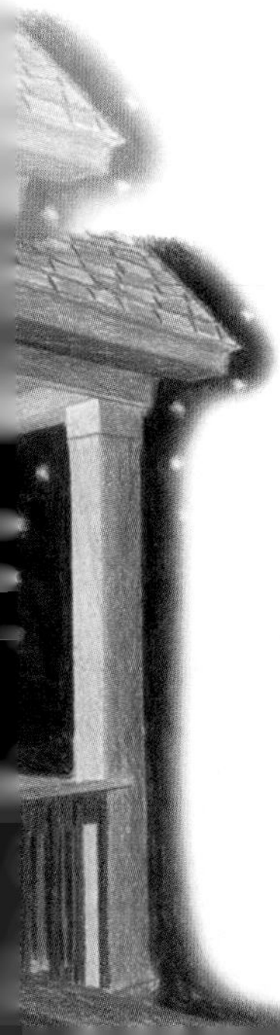

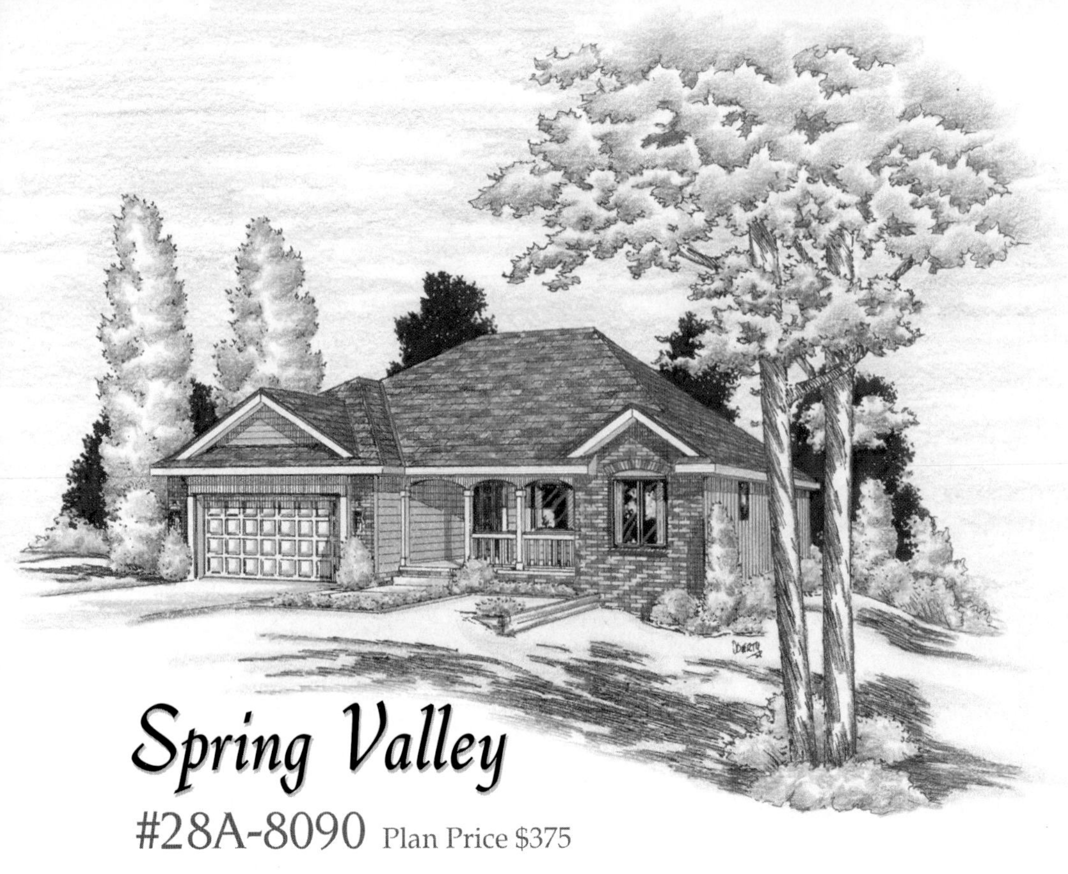

Spring Valley

#28A-8090 Plan Price $375

Total Square Feet: 1453 Sq. Ft.

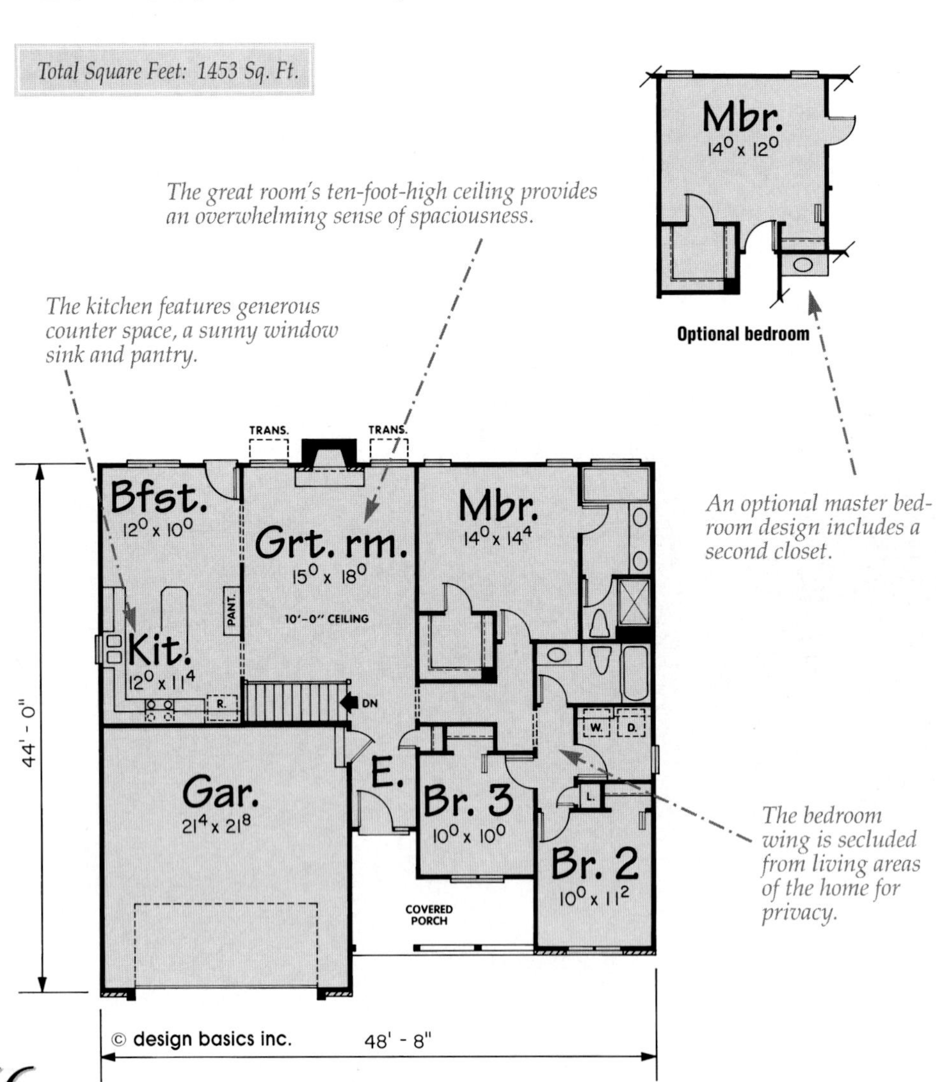

Our winter picnics on the living room floor – the complete feasts of hot dogs, baked beans, Jell-O and potato chips in the dead of a winter storm.

An in-between where the wind still rushes clean through the trees in our yard and the ice cream parlor is within a short drive. Where I live simply with my husband in our empty-nest years. Where my windows are shammy-clean and the floors are scrubbed on hand and knee. And where clothes come in fresh off our backyard clothesline.

As simplistic as they seem, she would even be proud of the new traditions I've forged: Our winter picnics on the living room floor – the complete feasts of hot dogs baked beans, Jell-O and potato chips in the dead of a winter storm. The Saturday wash day instead of Monday. The macaroni and cheese parties. My child-care career.

And maybe she would understand, as I do, that a place – if you've lived there long enough – becomes a part of you. And that no matter how hard we try, there's nothing that can change it. That we wouldn't be quite the person we are without the ritual of our homes. And yet, as often as we can, we dream our city-girl dreams, always reinventing ourselves and our home. Always remaining a part of what we were.

design basics inc. HOME PLAN DESIGN SERVICE

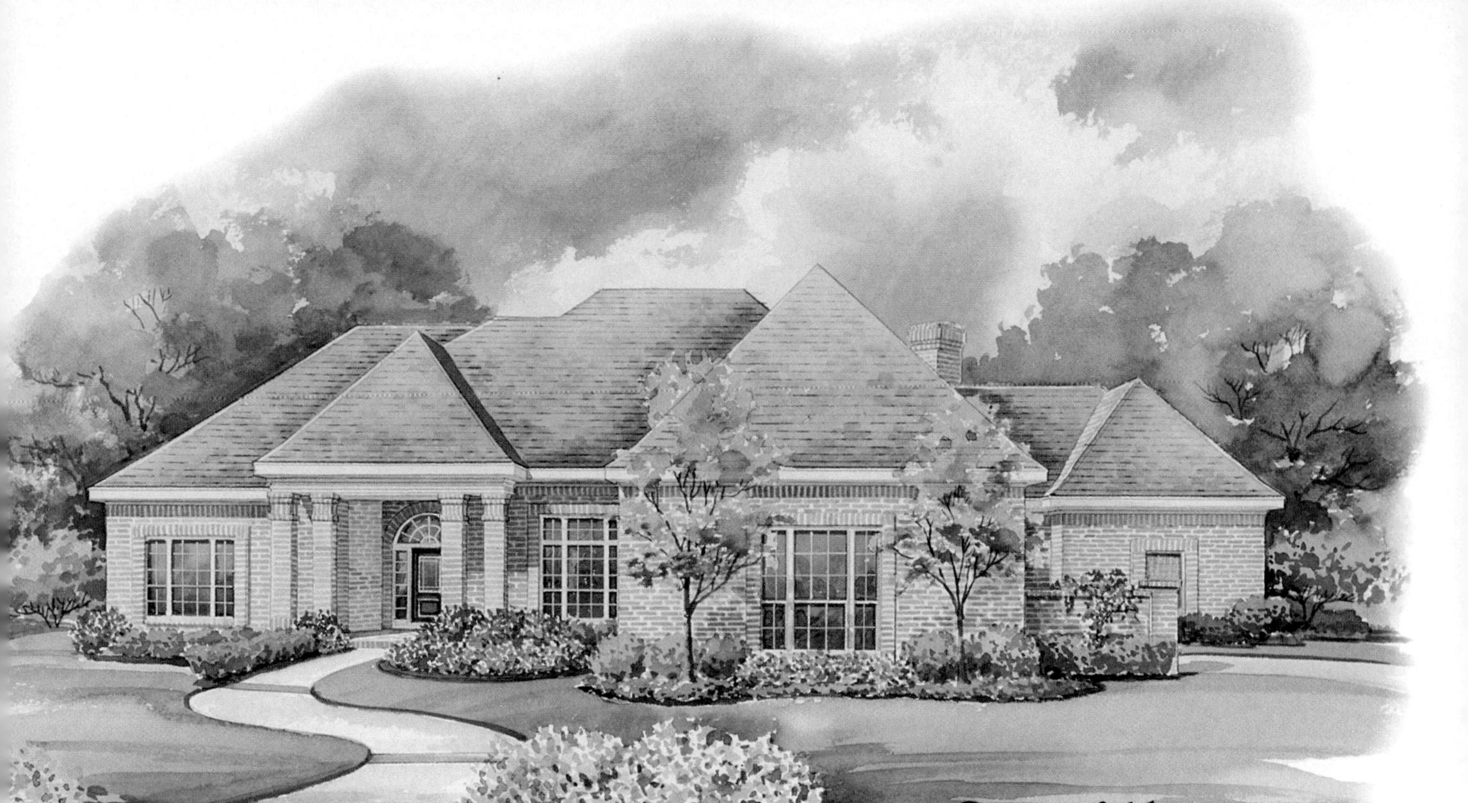

The Whitmore

#28A-9120 Plan Price $730

Total Square Feet: 3312 Sq. Ft.

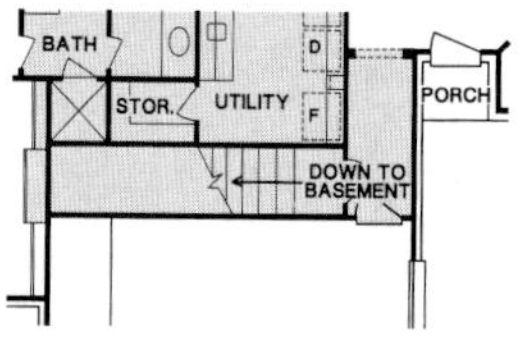

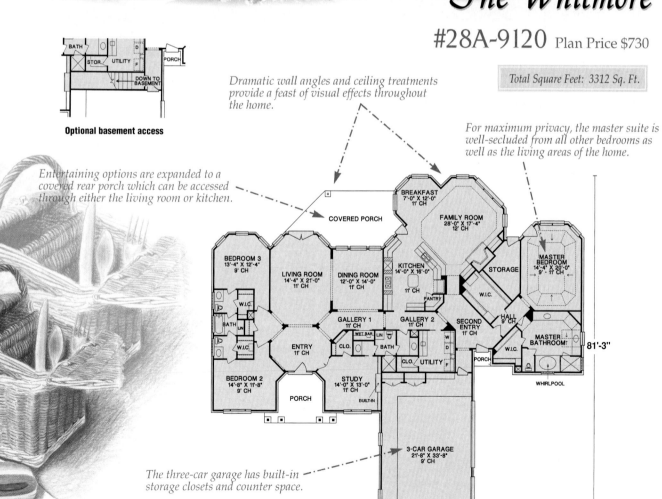

Optional basement access

Dramatic wall angles and ceiling treatments provide a feast of visual effects throughout the home.

For maximum privacy, the master suite is well-secluded from all other bedrooms as well as the living areas of the home.

Entertaining options are expanded to a covered rear porch which can be accessed through either the living room or kitchen.

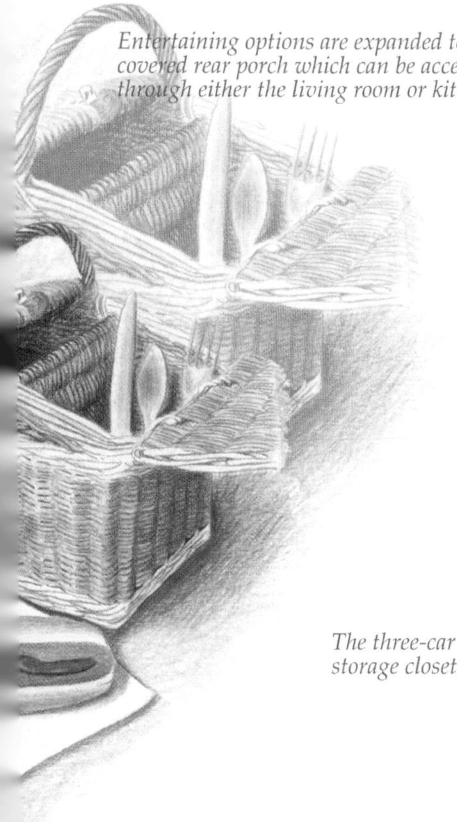

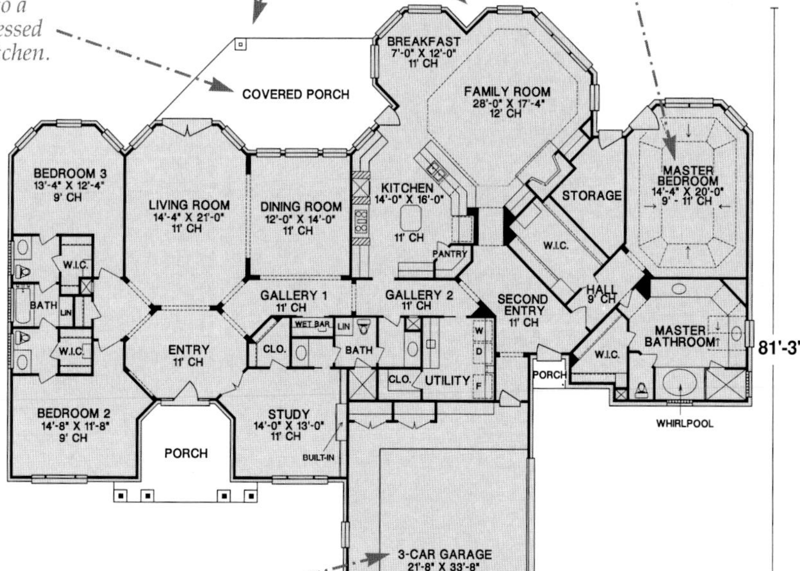

The three-car garage has built-in storage closets and counter space.

BATH STOR. UTILITY D F PORCH DOWN TO BASEMENT

BREAKFAST 7'-0" X 12'-0" 11' CH
FAMILY ROOM 28'-0" X 17'-4" 12' CH
COVERED PORCH
BEDROOM 3 13'-4" X 12'-4" 9' CH
LIVING ROOM 14'-4" X 21'-0" 11' CH
DINING ROOM 12'-0" X 14'-0" 11' CH
KITCHEN 14'-0" X 16'-0" 11' CH
PANTRY
STORAGE
MASTER BEDROOM 14'-4" X 20'-0" 9' - 11' CH
W.I.C.
HALL 9' CH
GALLERY 1 11' CH
GALLERY 2 11' CH
SECOND ENTRY 11' CH
BATH LIN W.I.C.
ENTRY 11' CH
CLO. WET BAR LIN BATH
CLO. UTILITY W D F
PORCH
MASTER BATHROOM
W.I.C.
WHIRLPOOL
BEDROOM 2 14'-8" X 11'-8" 9' CH
PORCH
STUDY 14'-0" X 13'-0" 11' CH
BUILT-IN
3-CAR GARAGE 21'-8" X 33'-8" 9' CH
81'-3"
90'-11"

© CARMICHAEL & DAME DESIGNS, INC.

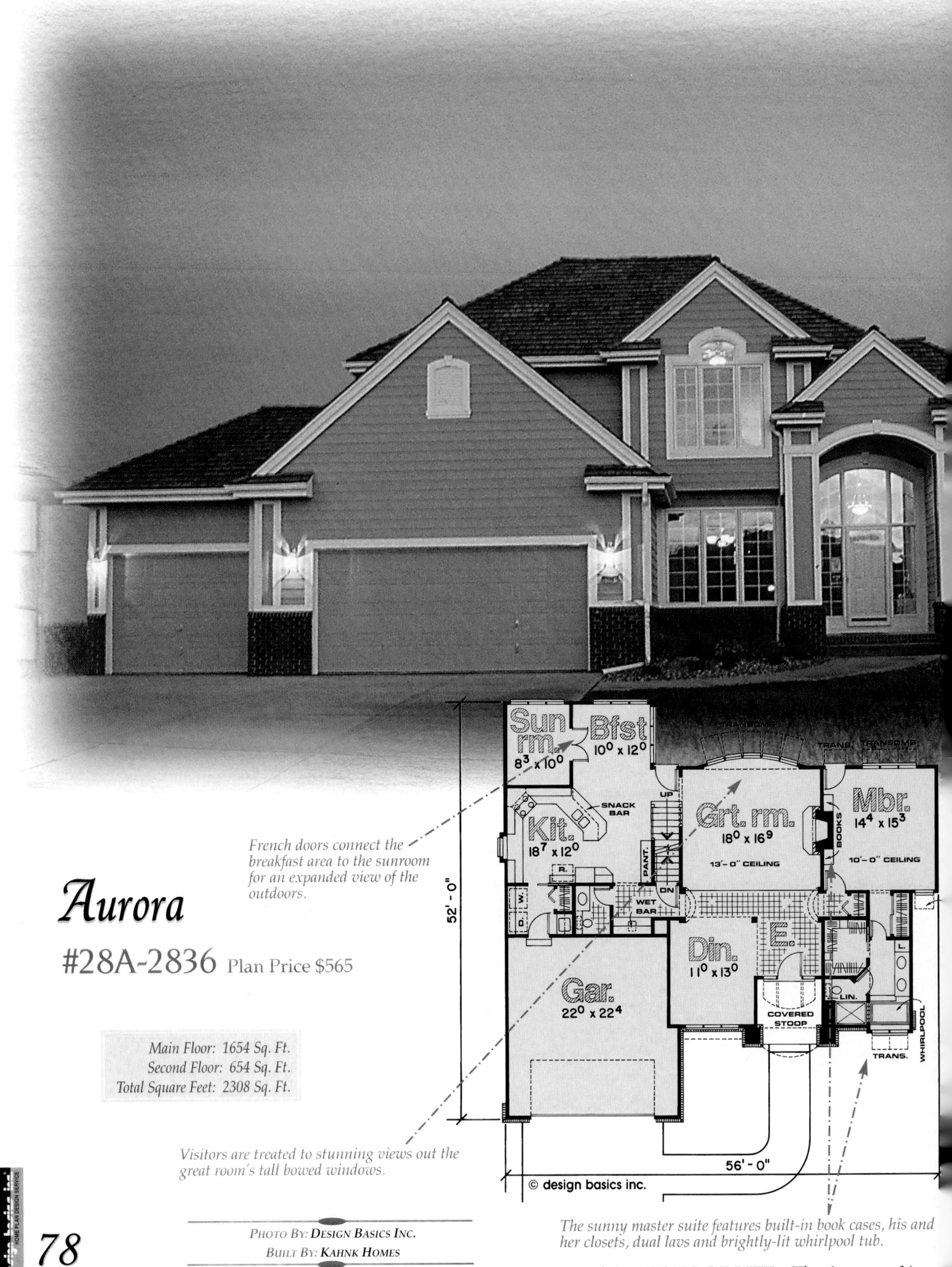

French doors connect the breakfast area to the sunroom for an expanded view of the outdoors.

Aurora

#28A-2836 Plan Price $565

Main Floor: 1654 Sq. Ft.
Second Floor: 654 Sq. Ft.
Total Square Feet: 2308 Sq. Ft.

Visitors are treated to stunning views out the great room's tall bowed windows.

The sunny master suite features built-in book cases, his and her closets, dual lavs and brightly-lit whirlpool tub.

PHOTO BY: DESIGN BASICS INC.
BUILT BY: KAHNK HOMES

The home in the photograph may have been altered from the original plan.

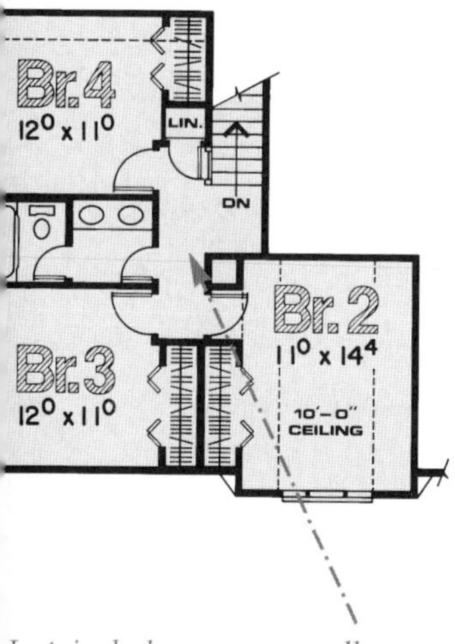

Ipstairs bedrooms are equally ospitable to guests from out-of- own, or kids home from college.

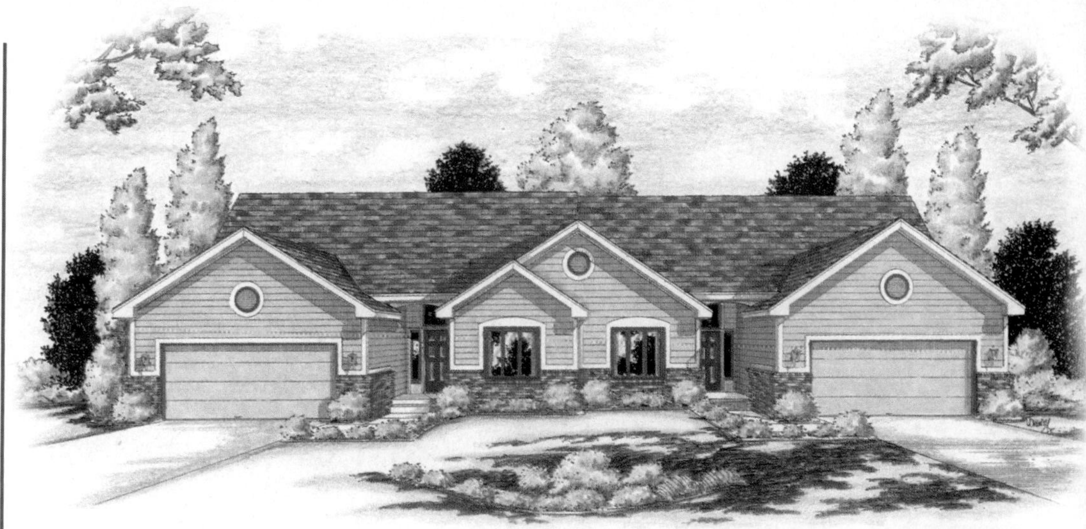

Duplex Plan

#28A-4628 Plan Price $595

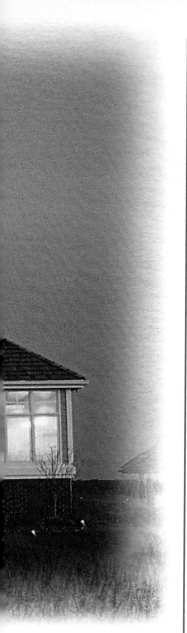

ADDITIONAL DUPLEX PLANS
are available from Design Basics. Call 1-800-947-7526 for information.

A 3-sided fireplace warms the atmosphere of the great room and breakfast area.

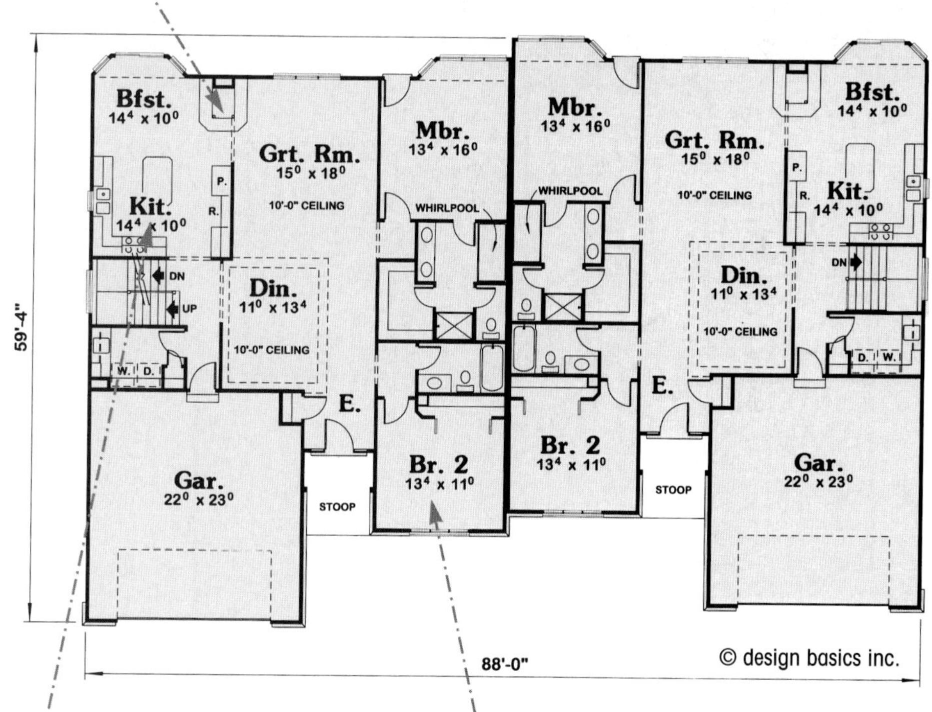

The island kitchen offers plenty of space for the serious cook and is only steps away from the formal dining room

Bedroom #2 is adjacent to a full bath and can easily opt as a den or home office.

LEFT SIDE
First Level: 1685 Sq. Ft.
Second Level: 576 Sq. Ft.
Total Square Feet: 2261 Sq. Ft.

RIGHT SIDE
Finished Sq. Ft. 1685

Br. 3
12^0 x 13^0
Br. 4
12^0 x 13^0
DN

Third and fourth bedrooms welcome out-of-town guests and colllege students home for the holidays.

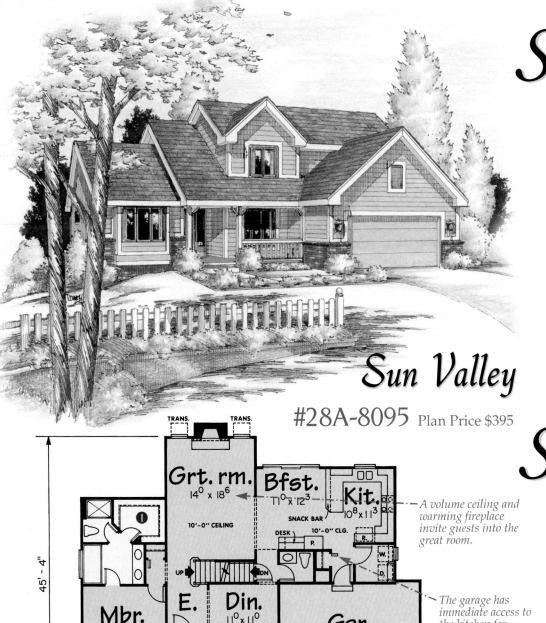

Sun Valley

#28A-8095 Plan Price $395

Grt. rm. $14^0 \times 18^6$
10'-0" CEILING
Bfst. $11^0 \times 12^3$
SNACK BAR
DESK
10'-0" CLG.
Kit. $10^8 \times 11^3$
Mbr. $13^0 \times 15^0$
E.
Din. $11^0 \times 11^0$
Gar. $22^0 \times 22^4$
COVERED PORCH
TRANS.
45' - 4"
54' - 0"

© design basics inc.

A volume ceiling and warming fireplace invite guests into the great room.

The garage has immediate access to the kitchen for unloading groceries.

Main Floor: 1298 Sq. Ft.
Second Floor: 396 Sq. Ft.
Total Square Feet: 1694 Sq. Ft.

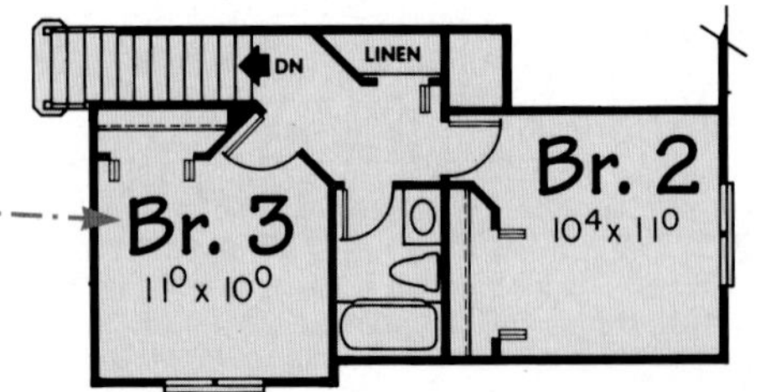

Two second-floor bedrooms are secluded from the master suite and activity on the main floor.

SITUATION

My husband and I are definitely not morning people. And when we get ready for work, nothing is more annoying than our tight bathroom. Many years of being together has taught us to give each other our space – even when we're both running late. But we both agree that our next home will need a bathroom with a lot of room, especially around the vanity area. .

SOLUTION

Plenty of space is a benefit of the master baths in both the Sun Valley and Montgomery. With ample depth between the vanity and soaking tub in the Sun Valley, there's plenty of room to get dressed while the spouse shaves or puts on make-up (❶, at left). The master bath in the Montgomery, pictured here, features six feet of depth from the vanity along with decorative arches and French doors (❷, at right).

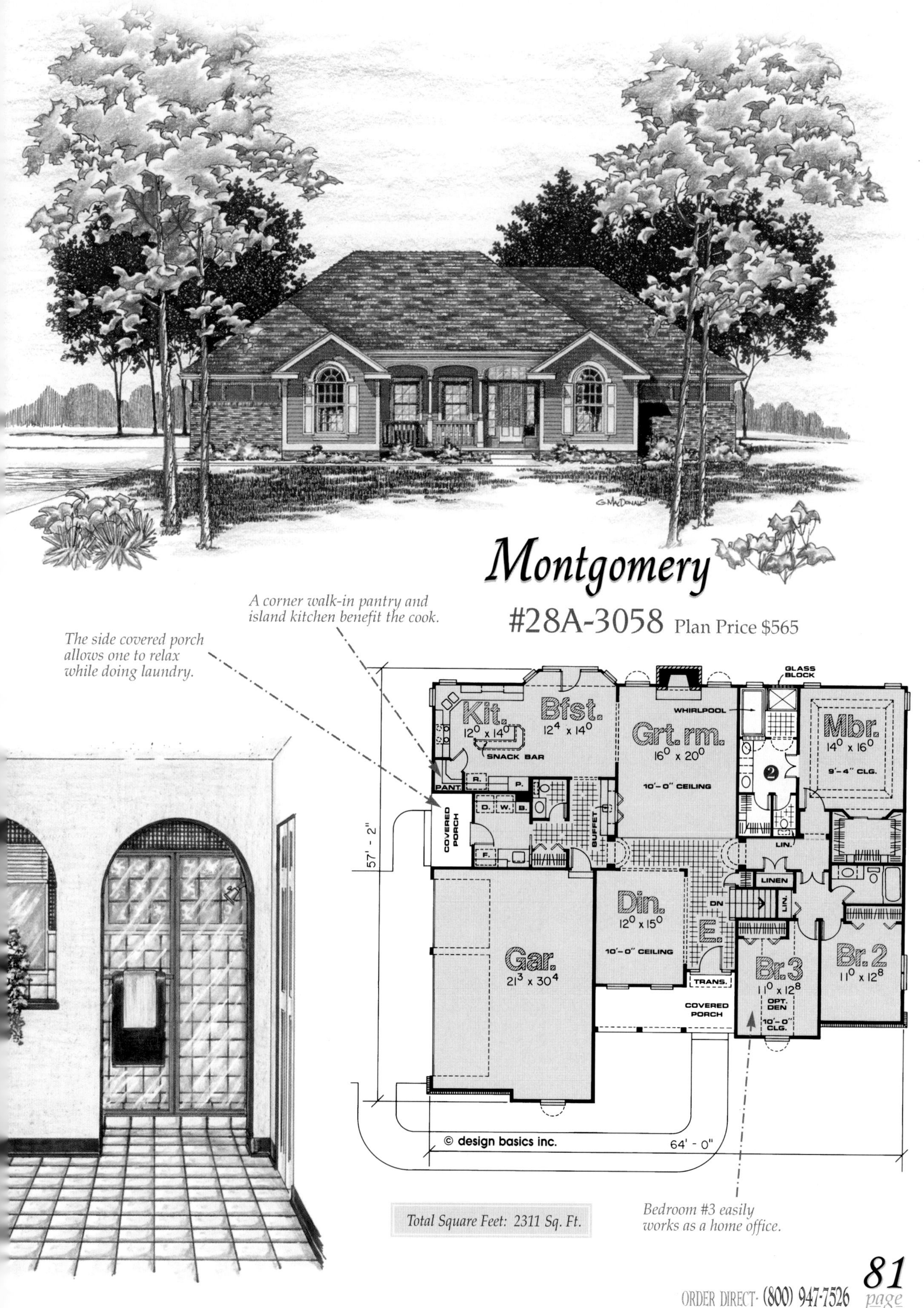

© design basics inc.

Montgomery

#28A-3058 Plan Price $565

A corner walk-in pantry and island kitchen benefit the cook.

The side covered porch allows one to relax while doing laundry.

Bedroom #3 easily works as a home office.

Total Square Feet: 2311 Sq. Ft.

SITUATION

Now that the kids have been gone for a number of years, we've gotten used to quiet, contemplative time, especially around bedtime and in the morning. But when they come home with the grandkids, it's sometimes hard to get a good night's rest when they sleep in nearby bedrooms. (I forgot how much work young children are!) Because of this I need a home with guest bedrooms that are located in a different part of the house from our bedroom. . .

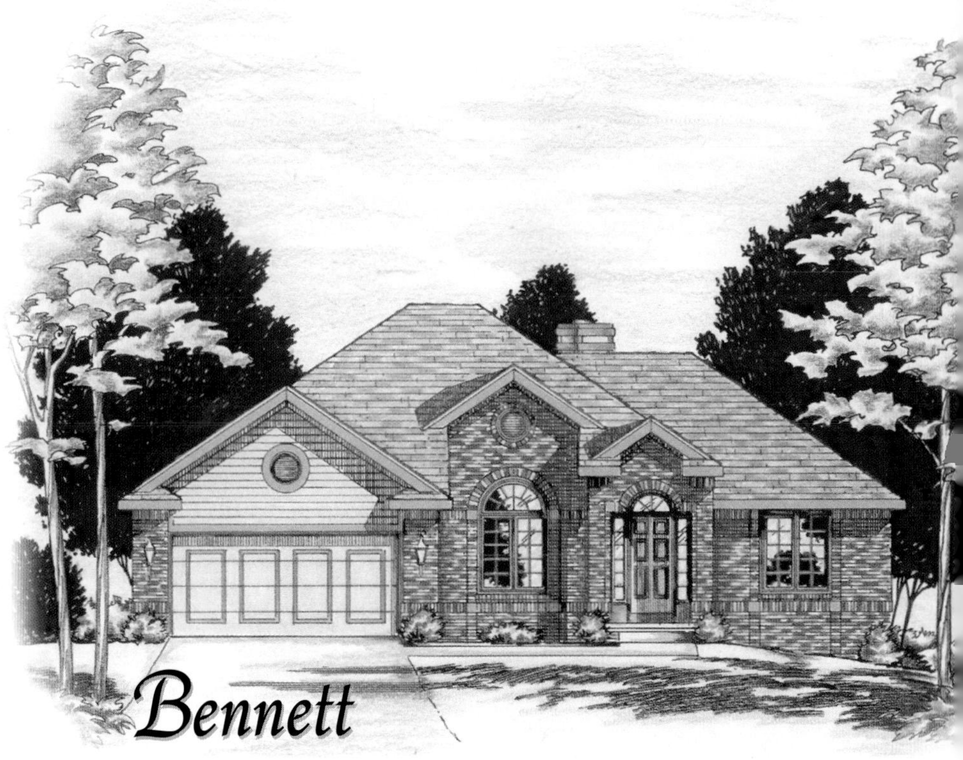

#28A-3577 Plan Price $505

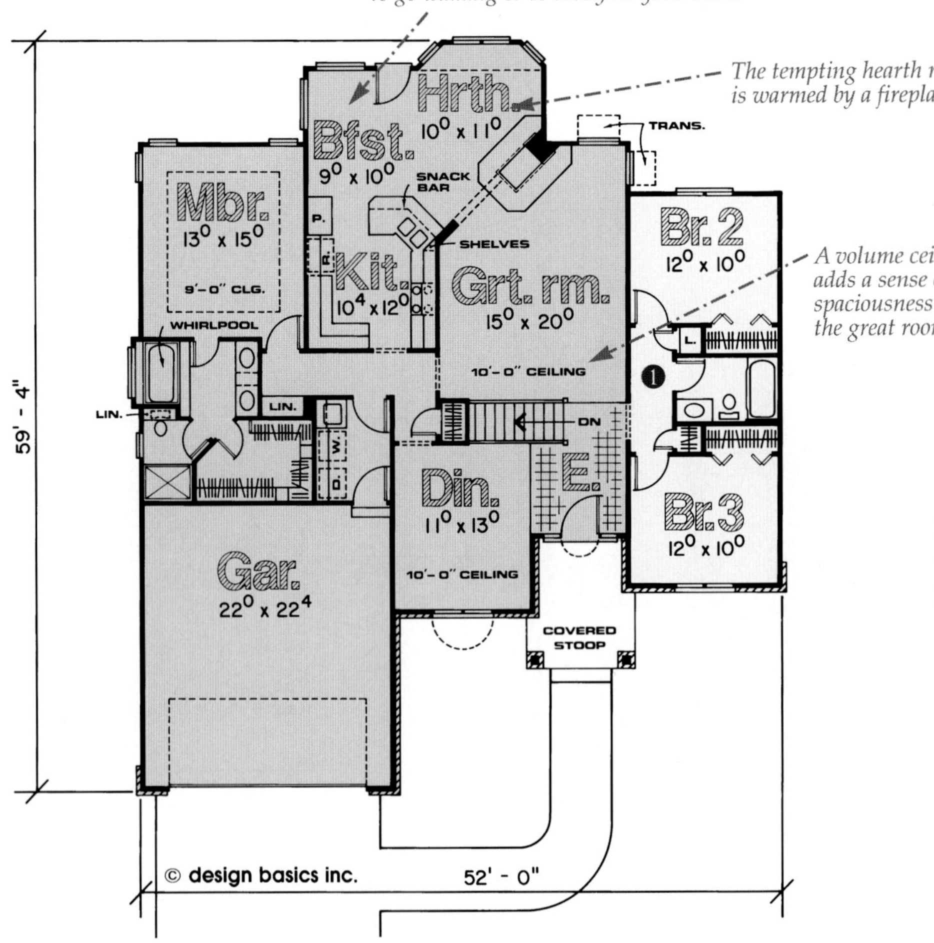

SOLUTION

The one-story Bennett offers two secondary bedrooms that are secluded from the master suite by the living areas of the home (❶, at right). In the Timber Point, three bedrooms, secluded on the second floor, are also located on the opposite end of the home providing maximum privacy to the master suite (❷, at far right).

Total Square Feet: 1782 Sq. Ft.

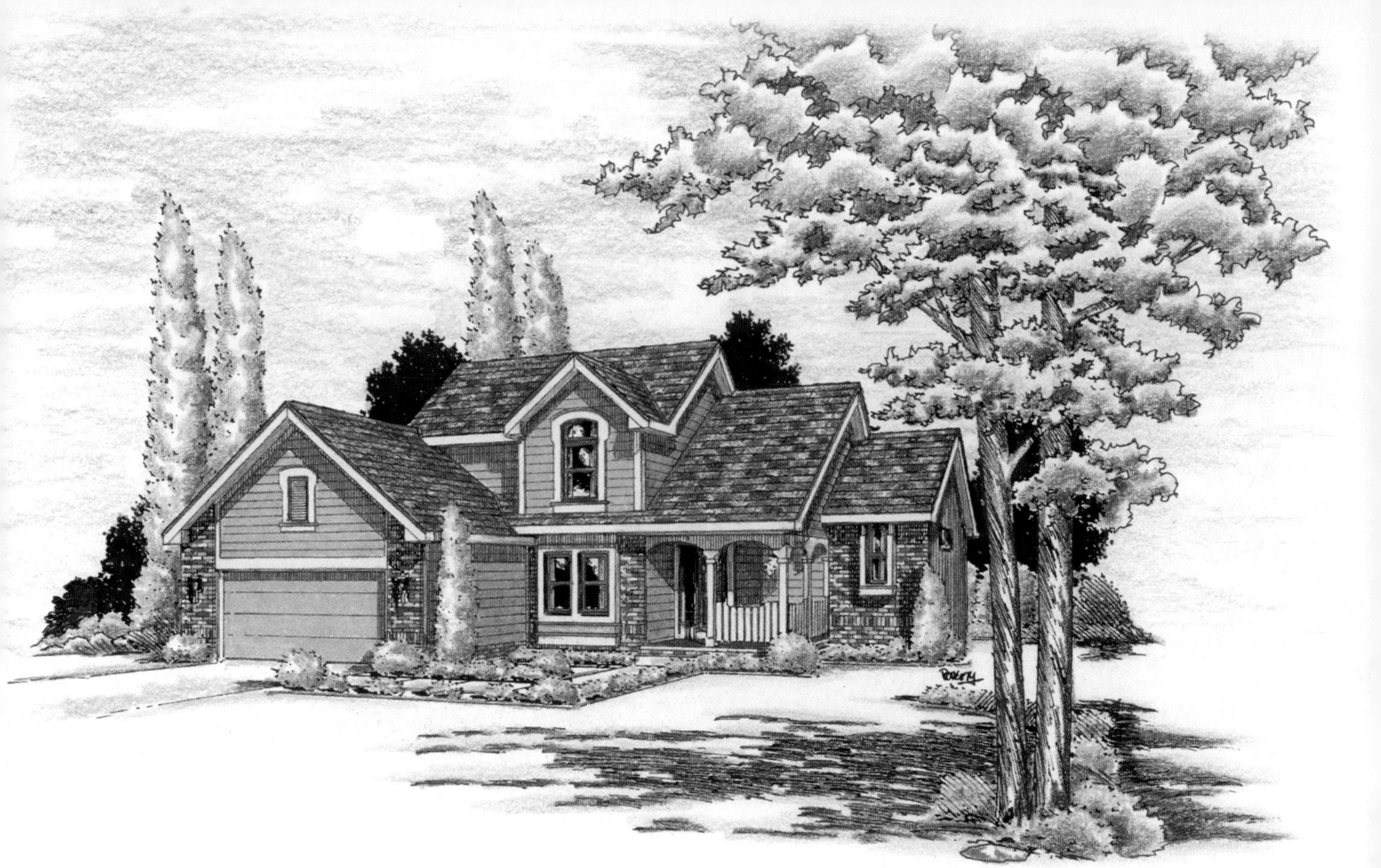

Timber Point

#28A-8075 Plan Price $425

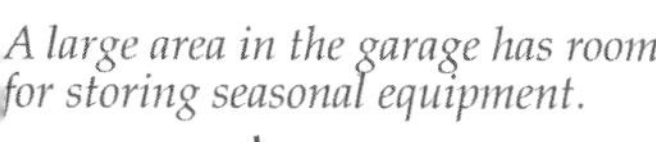

A large area in the garage has room for storing seasonal equipment.

A built-in desk provides a place for a home computer.

A pampering master bath offers a convenient dual-lav vanity and a soaking tub to relax in.

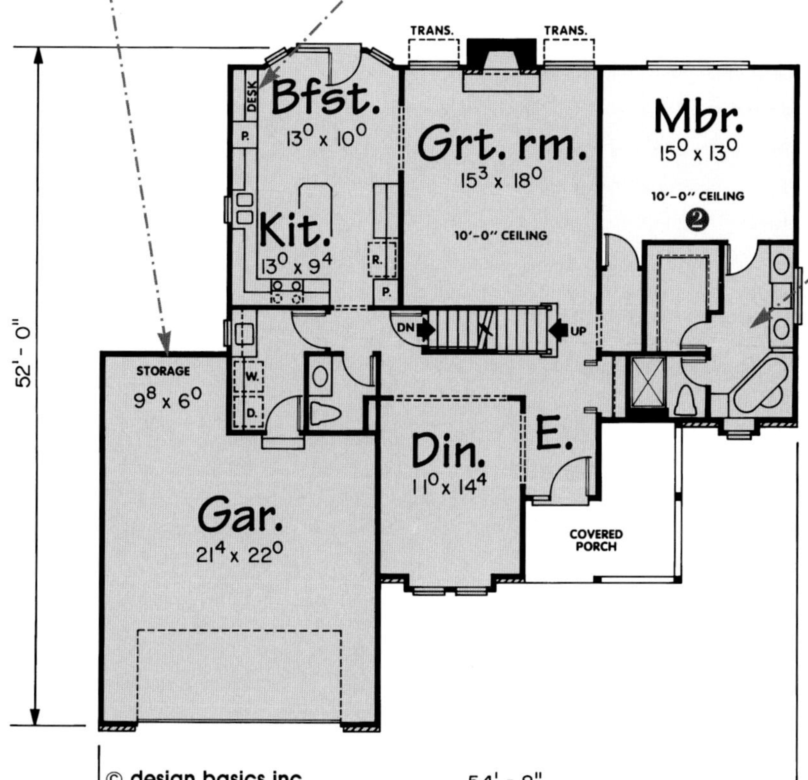

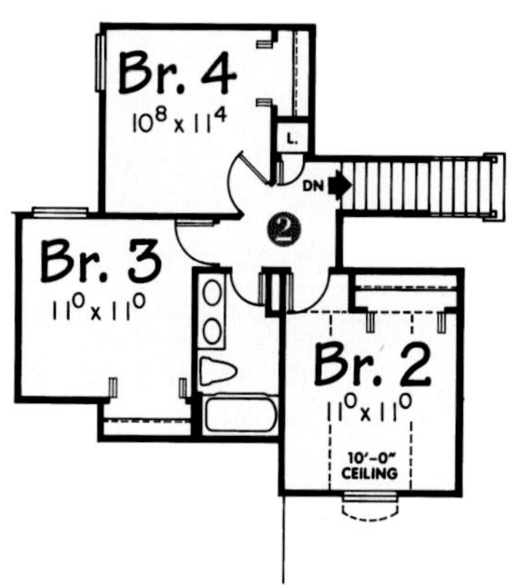

Main Floor: 1426 Sq. Ft.
Second Floor: 568 Sq. Ft.
Total Square Feet: 1994 Sq. Ft.

COPYRIGHT
Cans & Cannots

ALL DESIGN BASICS PLANS HAVE BEEN REGISTERED
ORIGINAL
C
DRAFT
WITH THE U.S. COPYRIGHT OFFICE

These days, it seems almost everybody has a question about what can or cannot be done with copyrighted home plans. At Design Basics, we know US copyright law can sometimes get complex and confusing, but here are a few of the basic points of the law you'll want to remember.

Once you've purchased a plan from us and have received a Design Basics construction license,

You Can . . .

- Construct the plan as originally designed, or change it to meet your specific needs.
- Build it as many times as you wish *without* additional reuse fees.
- Make duplicate blueprint copies as needed for construction.

You Cannot . . .

- Build our plans without a Design Basics construction license.
- Copy *any* part of our original designs to create another design of your own.
- Claim copyright on changes you make to our plans.
- Give a plan to someone else for construction purposes.
- Sell the plan.

PROTECT YOUR RIGHTS

to build, modify and reproduce our home plans with a Design Basics construction license.

CONSTRUCTION LICENS

as original purchaser of plan number

is hereby granted a non-transferable, non-exclusive license to build the home depicted in this plan and is given the right to reproduce this plan only as required for such construction. No re-use fee is required if the original purchaser builds this home more than once. Permission is also given to make modifications to this plan, but no permission is given to claim copyright on the original or any derivative works of this plan. No other rights are granted and any further distribution is strictly prohibited.

Signed

Date

License Number

RETAIN IN YOUR FILES FOR FUTURE REFERENCE

Valid when the official Gold Seal™ is embossed above.

11112 John Galt Boulevard Omaha, Nebraska 68137 Toll Free 800-947-PLAN 402-331-9223 FAX 402-331-5507

design basics inc. HOME PLAN DESIGN SERVICE

The above points are provided as general guidelines only. Additional information is provided with each home plan purchase, or is available upon request at (800) 947-7526.

CUSTOMIZED PLAN CHANGES

PRICE SCHEDULE

2 X 6 EXTERIOR WALLS .... $150 .....
FROM STANDARD 2 X 4 TO 2 X 6 EXTERIOR WALLS

EACH GARAGE ALTERATION .... $275 .....
- FRONT-ENTRY TO SIDE LOAD (OR VICE VERSA)
- 2-CAR TO 3-CAR (OR VICE VERSA)
- 2-CAR FRONT-ENTRY TO 3-CAR SIDE -LOAD (OR VICE VERSA)
- 3-CAR FRONT-ENTRY TO 2-CAR SIDE -LOAD (OR VICE VERSA)

WALK-OUT BASEMENT .... $175 .....

CRAWL SPACE FOUNDATION .... $225 .....

SLAB FOUNDATION .... $225 .....

STRETCH CHANGES .... $5 per lineal foot of cut

ADDITIONAL BRICK TO SIDES & REAR .... $325 .....

ADDITIONAL BRICK TO FRONT, SIDES AND REAR .... $425 .....

ALTERNATE PRELIMINARY ELEVATION .... $150 .....

9-FOOT MAIN LEVEL WALLS .... starting at $150

SPECIFY WINDOW BRAND .... $95 .....

POURED CONCRETE FOUNDATION .... $25 .....
ONLY WITH OTHER CHANGES

ADDING ONE COURSE (8") TO THE FOUNDATION HEIGHT
ONLY WITH OTHER CHANGES .... $25 .....

NOTE

- All plan changes come to you on erasable, reproducible vellums.
- An unchanged set of original vellums is available for only $50 along with your plan changes.
- Gold Seal™ changes are not made to the artist's renderings, electrical, sections or cabinets.
- Prices are subject to change.

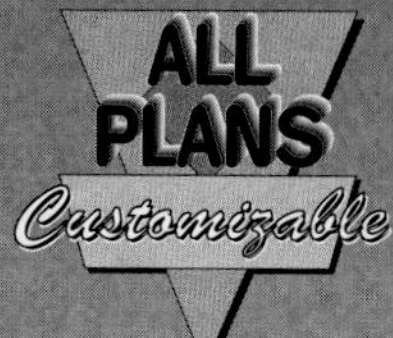

As a part of our commitment to help you achieve the "perfect" home, we offer an extensive variety of plan changes for any Design Basics plan. For those whose decision to purchase a home plan is contingent upon the feasibility of a plan change, our Customer Support Specialists will, in most cases, be able to provide a FREE price quote for the changes.

call us toll-free at

(800) 947-7526

to order plan changes listed here, or if you have questions regarding plan changes not listed.

DISCOVER

MORE ABOUT DESIGN BASICS ON THE

WORLD WIDE WEB

www.designbasics.com

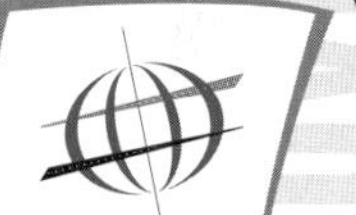

More Photographed Home Plan Designs · *Useful information about our Products and Services* · *Commonly Asked Questions about Building a New Home* · *Details about Design Basics Construction Prints* · *Custom Change Information* · *What's New from Design Basics* · *All About Design Basics*

E-MAIL dbi@synergy.net

PLANS TO BUILD?

1. Gold Seal™ Home Plan Book Set. 442 of today's most sought-after one-story, 1½ and 2-story home plan ideas.

$19.95 each. SPECIAL OFFER – Order the set of 5 for $84.95.

Homes of Distinction – 86 plans under 1800'
Homes of Sophistication – 106 plans, 1800' - 2199'
Homes of Elegance – 107 plans, 2200' - 2599'
Homes of Prominence – 75 plans, 2600' - 2999'
Homes of Grandeur – 68 plans, 3000' - 4000'

2. Timeless Legacy™, A Collection of Fine Home Designs by Carmichael & Dame. 52 breathtaking luxury home designs from 3300' to 4500'. Includes artful rear views of each home.

Available for $25

3. Heartland Home Plans™. 120 plan ideas designed for every-day practicality. Warm, unpretentious elevations easily adapt to individual lifestyles.

Just $8.95

4. The Narrow Book™. 217 one-story, 1½ story and 2-story home plans that are from 26 to 50 feet wide. Many can be joined together to create customized duplex plans.

Just $14.95

5. On the Porch™ – *A Designer's Journal of Notes and Sketches.* 64 designs from Gold Seal™, Heartland Home Plans™ and Timeless Legacy™ – each one with a porch. Includes essays on the porch and its role in traditional design.

Only $2.95

6. Photographed Portraits of an American Home™. 100 of our finest designs, beautifully photographed and tastefully presented among nostalgic photo album memories of "home". A must for any sales center's coffee-table.

Only $14.95

7. Easy Living One-Story Designs™. 155 one-story home designs from the Gold Seal™, Heartland Home Plans™ and Timeless Legacy™ collections, together in one plan book.

Just $7.95

Please include $2.95 Shipping & Handling when ordering one plan book, or $4.95 when ordering 2 or more plan books.

• All book sales subject to availability •

design basics inc.
HOME PLAN DESIGN SERVICE
11112 John Galt Blvd Omaha, NE 68137-2384

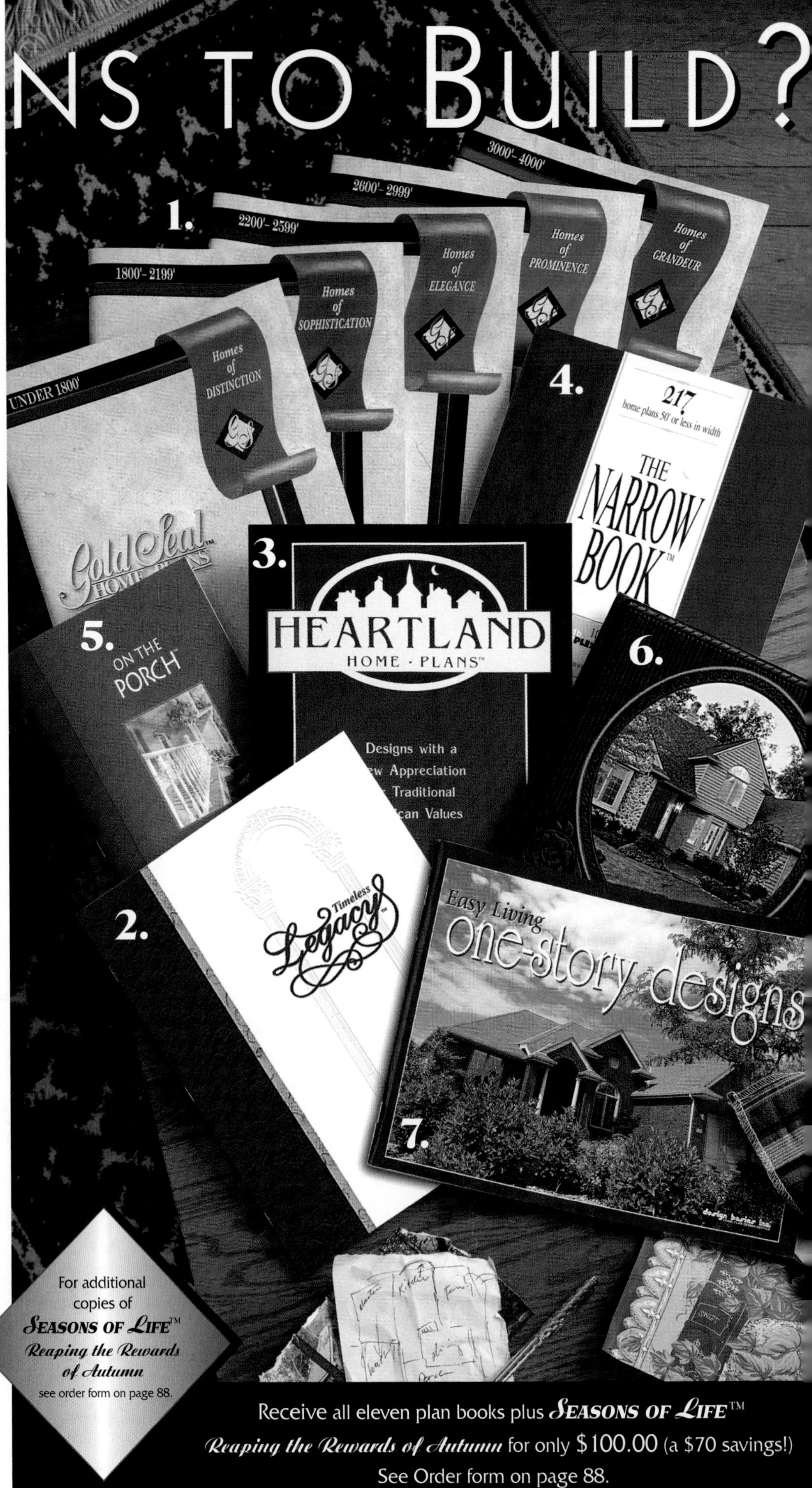

For additional copies of *Seasons of Life*™ *Reaping the Rewards of Autumn* see order form on page 88.

Receive all eleven plan books plus *Seasons of Life*™ *Reaping the Rewards of Autumn* for only $100.00 (a $70 savings!) See Order form on page 88.

I LOVE this floor plan but . . .

I WANT TO SEE THE HOME IN MORE DETAIL BEFORE I BUY THE PLANS.

HOW DOES IT LOOK FROM ALL SIDES?

WILL MY GRANDMA'S HUTCH FIT?

WILL I NEED TO ALTER THE ROOM SIZES?

We understand that comprehending the finished home from a set of floor plans is a challenge. Our Study Print & Furniture Layout Guide™ was designed to help you better understand how your Design Basics' home will "live." This helpful home planning tool comes with a Study Print showing views of all exterior elevations and aerial views of the roof. It also includes the Furniture Layout Guide™, made up of a 1/4" scale floor plan and over 100 reusable furniture pieces allowing you to plan furniture placement and determine adequate room sizes. The Study Print & Furniture Layout Guide is available for any Design Basics' home plan.

Order today by calling (800) 947-7526.

The Study Print & Furniture Layout Guide™ Only $29.95

A Plan From Design Basics: What's In It For You?

Plans come to you on high-quality reproducible vellums and include the following:

1. Cover Page. Each Design Basics home plan features the rendered elevation and informative reference sections including: general notes and design criteria;* abbreviations; and symbols for your Design Basics' plan.

2. Elevations. Drafted at 1/4" scale for the front and 1/8" scale for the rear and sides. All elevations are detailed and an aerial view of the roof is provided, showing all hips, valleys and ridges.

3. Foundations. Drafted at 1/4" scale. Block foundations and basements are standard. We also show the HVAC equipment, structural information,* steel beam and pole locations and the direction and spacing of the floor system above.

4. Main Level Floor Plan. 1/4" scale. Fully dimensioned from stud to stud for ease of framing. 2"x4" walls are standard. The detailed drawings include such things as structural header locations, framing layout and kitchen layout.

5. Second Level Floor Plan. 1/4" scale. Dimensioned from stud to stud and drafted to the same degree of detail as the main level floor plan.*

6. Interior Elevations. Useful for the cabinet and bidding process, this page shows all kitchen and bathroom cabinets as well as any other cabinet elevations.

7. Electrical and Sections. Illustrated on a separate page for clarity, the el cal plan shows suggested electrical layout for the found main and second level floor plans. Typical wall, canti stair, brick and fireplace sections are provided to fu explain construction of these areas.

All plan orders received prior to 2:00 p.m. CT will be proce inspected and shipped out the same afternoon via 2nd busines air within the continental United States. All other product orders will b via UPS ground service. Full Technical Support is available for any plan pur from Design Basics. Our Technical Support Specialists provide unlimited tec support free of charge and answer questions regarding construction methods, ing techniques and more. Please call 800-947-7526 for more information.

CONSTRUCTION LICENSE

When you purchase a Design Basics home plan, you receive a Construction Li which gives you certain rights in building the home depicted in that plan, inclu

No Re-Use Fee. As the original purchaser of a Design Basics home pla Construction License permits you to build the plan as many times as you lik

Local Modifications. The Construction License allows you to make mo tions to your Design Basics plans. We offer a complete custom change servi you may have the desired changes done locally by a qualified draftsman, d er, architect or engineer.

Running Blueprints. Your plans are sent to you on vellum paper that repro well on your blueprint machine. The Construction License authorizes you c blueprint facility, at your direction, to make as many copies of the plan fro vellum masters as you need for construction purposes.

* Our plans are drafted to meet average conditions and codes in the state of Nebraska, at the time they are designed. Because codes and requirements can change and may vary from jurisdiction to jurisdiction, Design Basics I not warrant compliance with any specific code or regulation. All Design Basics plans can be adapted to your local building codes and requirements. It is the responsibility of the purchaser and/or builder of each plan to see structure is built in strict compliance with all governing municipal codes (city, county, state and federal).

Order Via Mail or Fax - Attention Dept. 28A

✔	HOME PLAN PRODUCTS	PLAN NO.	QTY.	PRICE	SHIPPING & HANDLING	TOTAL
☐	1 Complete Set of Master Reproducible/Modifiable				No Charge	$
☐	Add'l. Sets of Blueprint Plan #9160, #9143 & #9				$4.95 or No Charge if Shipped with plan	$
☐	Add'l. Sets of Mirror Plan #9160, #9143 &				$4.95 or No Charge if Shipped with plan	$
☐	Materials & Estim (Not Available for pla				$4.95 or No Charge if Shipped with plan	$
☐	Study Print & Furnit *Study print (only) for plans				$4.95	$
☐	Seasons of Life™-Reaping th				$2.95	$
☐	Plan Book Deal plus Seasons of L				$4.95	$
BOOK NUMBER						
					Individual Plan Books $2.95	$
					2 or More Plan Books $4.95	$

• All orders payable in U.S. funds only. • Shipping prices for Continental U.S. only • No refunds or exchanges, please.
• All Design Basics plans come with a basement foundation. • Alternate foundations available through our Custom Change Dept.

All COD's must be paid by Certified Check,Cashier's Check or Money Order. (Additional $5.00 charge on COD Orders) $ 5.00

Subtotal $

TX Res. Add 6.25% Tax (on plan #9160, #9143 & #9120 only) NE Residents Add 6.5% Sales Tax $

Total $

TO ORDER DIRECT: Call 800-947-7526
Ask for Dept 28A
Monday - Friday
7:00 a.m. - 6:00 p.m. CST

CANADIAN 1969 1999 ORDER HOTLINE 1-800-561-4169 30th YEAR BLUEPRINTS

Fax your order any time: (402) 331-5507
Or mail to Design Basics Inc., 11112 John Galt Blvd. • Omaha, NE 68137

Company Name________

Name________

Address________
Packages cannot be shipped to a P.O. Box

City______ State______ Zip______

Above address is ☐ Business address ☐ Residence addres

Phone ( )______ Date______

☐ VISA ☐ AMEX
☐ MC ☐ Discover
☐ Check or Money Order Enclosed

All COD's must be paid by Certified Check, Cashier's Check or Money Order. (Additional $5.00 charge on COD Orders)

Ex

Signature________

PRICES SUBJECT TO CHANGE

CODE 28A-13

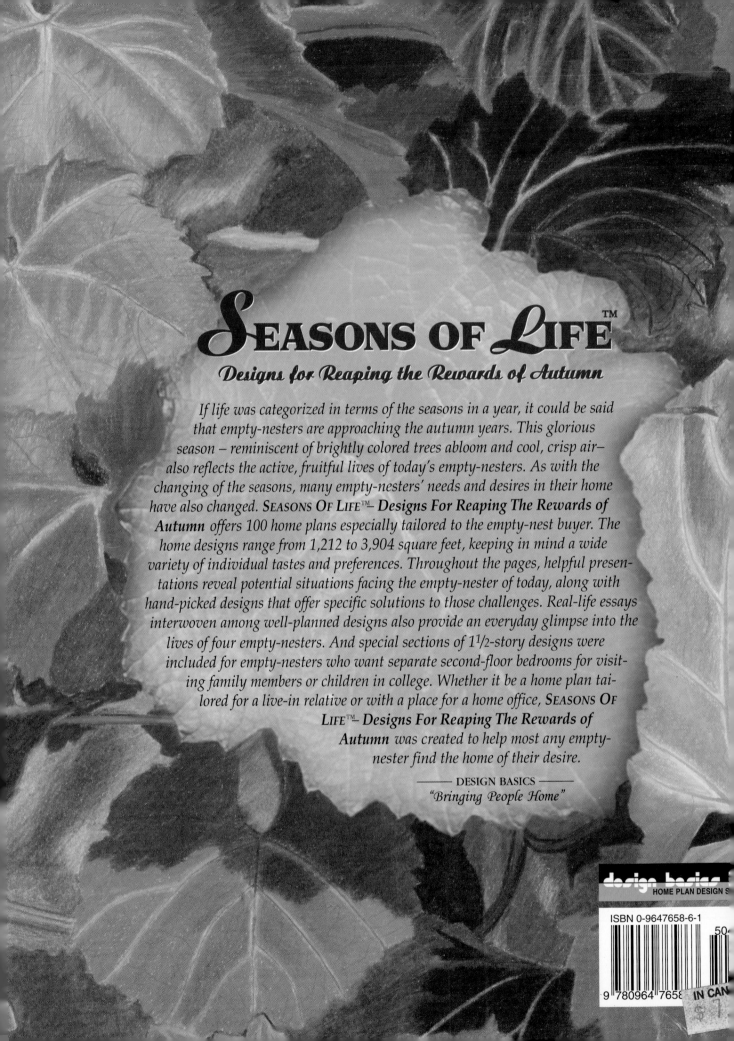

SEASONS OF LIFE™

Designs for Reaping the Rewards of Autumn

If life was categorized in terms of the seasons in a year, it could be said that empty-nesters are approaching the autumn years. This glorious season – reminiscent of brightly colored trees abloom and cool, crisp air– also reflects the active, fruitful lives of today's empty-nesters. As with the changing of the seasons, many empty-nesters' needs and desires in their home have also changed. **SEASONS OF LIFE™– Designs For Reaping The Rewards of Autumn** *offers 100 home plans especially tailored to the empty-nest buyer. The home designs range from 1,212 to 3,904 square feet, keeping in mind a wide variety of individual tastes and preferences. Throughout the pages, helpful presentations reveal potential situations facing the empty-nester of today, along with hand-picked designs that offer specific solutions to those challenges. Real-life essays interwoven among well-planned designs also provide an everyday glimpse into the lives of four empty-nesters. And special sections of 1½-story designs were included for empty-nesters who want separate second-floor bedrooms for visiting family members or children in college. Whether it be a home plan tailored for a live-in relative or with a place for a home office,* **SEASONS OF LIFE™– Designs For Reaping The Rewards of Autumn** *was created to help most any empty-nester find the home of their desire.*

——— DESIGN BASICS ———
"Bringing People Home"

design basics
HOME PLAN DESIGN S
ISBN 0-9647658-6-1
9 780964 7658
IN CAN
$ 7

design basics inc.®
HOME PLAN DESIGN SERVICE

SEASONS OF LIFE™

Designs for Living Summer's Journey

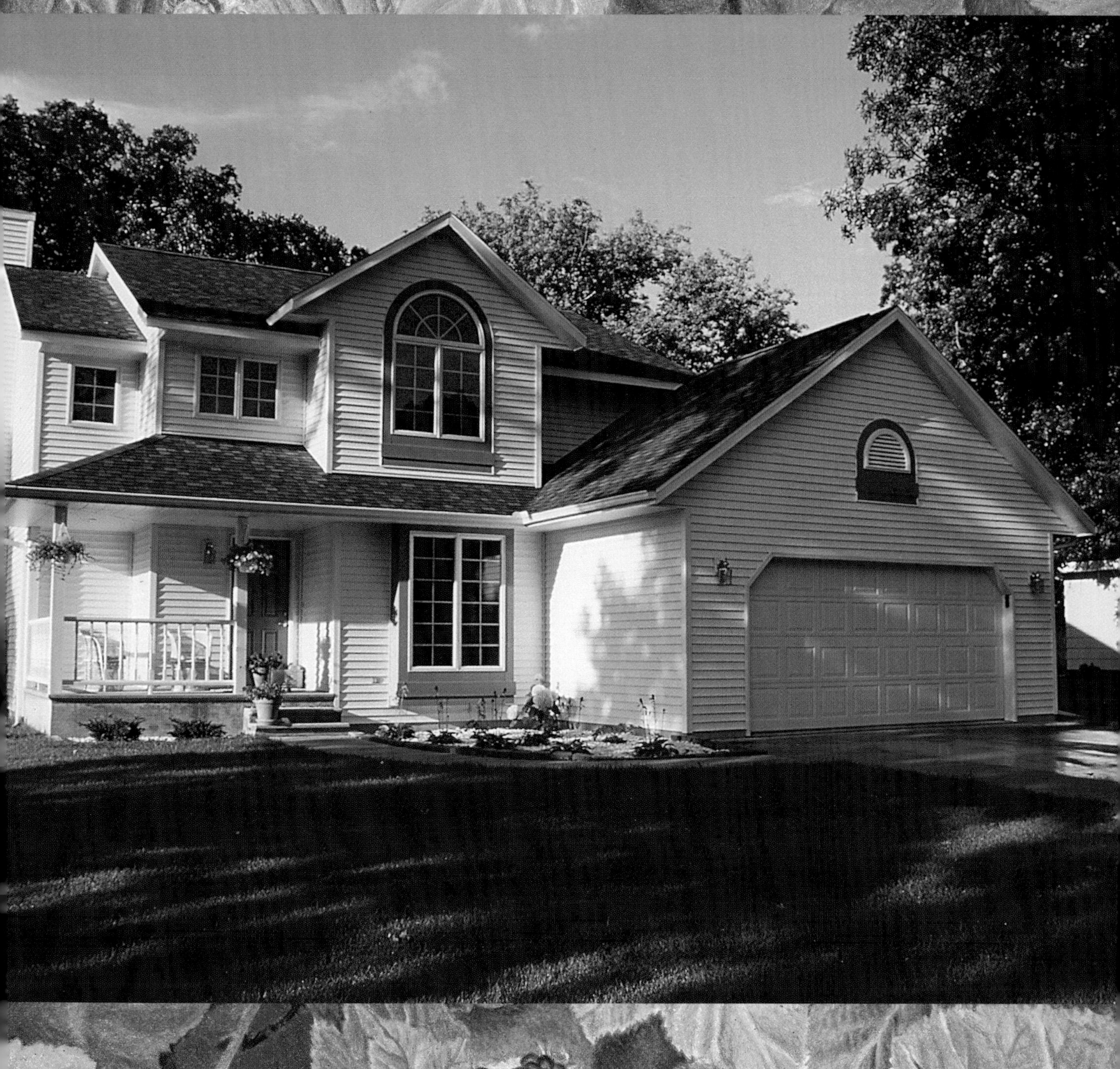

ONE HUNDRED HOME PLANS